Cleft Palate
Speech and Resonance

An Audio and Video Resource

Cleft Palate Speech and Resonance

An Audio and Video Resource

Linda D. Vallino, PhD

Head, Craniofacial Outcomes Research Laboratory/Senior Speech Scientist
Center for Pediatric Auditory and Speech Sciences
Nemours/Alfred I. duPont Hospital for Children
Clinical Professor of Pediatrics
Sidney Kimmel Medical College, Thomas Jefferson University
Adjunct Associate Professor, University of Delaware
Wilmington, Delaware

Dennis M. Ruscello, PhD

Professor of Communication Sciences and Disorders
Department of Communication Sciences and Disorders
College of Education and Human Services
Adjunct Professor of Otolaryngology
West Virginia University
Morgantown, West Virginia

David J. Zajac, PhD

Professor, Department of Dental Ecology
Adjunct Associate Professor, Division of Speech and Hearing Sciences
Department of Allied Health Sciences
University of North Carolina at Chapel Hill
Chapel Hill, North Carolina

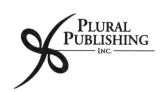

PLURAL
PUBLISHING
INC.

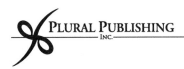

5521 Ruffin Road
San Diego, CA 92123

e-mail: information@pluralpublishing.com
website: http://www.pluralpublishing.com

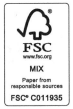

FSC
www.fsc.org
MIX
Paper from
responsible sources
FSC® C011935

Typeset in 10.5/13 Garamond Book by Flanagan's Publishing Services, Inc.
Printed in the United States of America by McNaughton & Gunn, Inc.
21 20 19   2 3 4 5

Library of Congress Cataloging-in-Publication Data

Names: Vallino, Linda D., author. | Ruscello, Dennis M., author. | Zajac,
   David J., author.
Title: Cleft palate speech and resonance : an audio and video resource /
   Linda D. Vallino, Dennis M. Ruscello, David J. Zajac.
Other titles: Complemented by (work): Evaluation and management of cleft lip
   and palate.
Description: San Diego, CA : Plural Publishing, Inc., [2019] | Developed to
   be a companion to the textbook: Evaluation and management of cleft lip and
   palate : a developmental perspective / David J. Zajac, Linda D. Vallino.
   2017. | Includes bibliographical references and index.
Identifiers: LCCN 2017058134| ISBN 9781635500233 (alk. paper) | ISBN
   1635500230 (alk. paper)
Subjects: | MESH: Cleft Palate | Velopharyngeal Insufficiency | Speech
   Disorders--prevention & control
Classification: LCC RD525 | NLM WV 440 | DDC 617.5/225--dc23
LC record available at https://lccn.loc.gov/2017058134

◼ Contents

◼ Preface

Cleft Palate Speech and Resonance: An Audio and Video Resource was developed to be a companion to the textbook, *Evaluation and Management of Cleft Lip and Palate: A Developmental Perspective* (Zajac & Vallino, 2017). It can also serve as a standalone text to facilitate learning about speech disorders associated with cleft palate (CP) and other problems of resonance in speakers without a cleft condition.

The original intent was to edit a series of digital audio and video samples for speech-language pathologists (SLPs) to use in becoming familiar with the speech, resonance, and phonatory characteristics of individuals with CP. That is, we wanted to create a clinical tool that would assist students and SLPs in developing their auditory perceptual identification skills. However, our discussions and literature searches over the past 2 years altered our thinking. The most pressing issue was that patients[1] with CP constitute a low-incidence population, and many clinicians have limited academic exposure and/or clinical training in this area, a shortcoming that many recognize. The result is that their knowledge base and clinical skills are limited. Grames (2008) provides an excellent discussion of the history of care of the individual with cleft palate in the United States, and she also identifies current issues that limit academic and clinical opportunities for students. Survey data collected by the American Speech-Language-Hearing Association (2012) and corroborated by others indicate that one of the significant challenges facing SLPs in the schools is the lack of education and training in low-incidence populations such as cleft palate (Bedwinek, 2007; Vallino, Lass, Bunnell, & Pannbacker, 2008).

The paradigm shift in our thinking resulted in the preparation of this *Resource.* The issues that currently prevail led us to alter our thinking in terms of developing a useful educational product for students and

---

[1]In this *Resource,* we use the word patient rather than client to refer to the speakers in the audio and video samples as they have all been managed by our respective hospital-based interdisciplinary teams. We acknowledge that community-based SLPs and those working in academic settings use the term client to refer to those individuals to whom they provide speech and language services.

clinicians. Rather than present a series of audio and video recordings that would only address a skill area, we decided to develop a publication that would address both knowledge and skill areas. While there are several excellent publications in the management of cleft lip and palate, we reasoned that both students and SLPs would benefit from a publication that focuses on cleft-related speech disorders with the opportunity to hear, see, and assess these disorders as well. The goals of this publication are to improve the knowledge base and clinical skills of students and SLPs by presenting current and evidence-based information and a range of auditory-perceptual experiences that will help them to identify the different speech, resonance, and phonatory problems associated in speakers with CP. It will also enable them to apply these concepts to care for the individual with cleft palate and interact with caregivers and cleft palate teams. Students and SLPs need easy access to information and materials, which explicitly deal with the particular communication disorder and are state of the art (Kuster, 2010). This is very important in cleft care, since assessment and treatment concepts have changed significantly over the past 25 years.

This *Resource* offers material for those who need such information and features a series of audio- and video-recorded speech samples and case studies that the student and practicing clinician can use to develop perceptual identification skills to assess patients with cleft palate and resonance disorders and also those with noncleft-related velopharyngeal dysfunction. The audio and video samples can be accessed on the PluralPlus companion website. For instructors, it can provide much-needed teaching materials that are necessary in the classroom, particularly where access to this population is limited. Practicing SLPs can also use it to retool their skills. Last, it can also be a great resource for dental and medical students, and residents who are learning about cleft palate.

The first chapter provides an overview of the velopharyngeal mechanism, followed by descriptions of resonance, articulation, and phonatory characteristics of speakers who have cleft palate. Hearing and other potential coexisting communication problems are also discussed. Chapter 2 focuses on a systematic assessment of communication problems associated with cleft palate. Chapter 3 provides an array of audio- and video-recorded speech samples and case examples illustrating a variety of speech problems associated with cleft palate, some of which may seem to be straightforward and others more complex. Here, the SLP will have an opportunity for independent practice in listening and analyzing these speech samples and to make recommendations for treatment, and to compare their analyses with ours provided in Appendices A and B. Because there are a variety of cases in which speech therapy is recommended, Chapter 4 describes treatment strategies to correct speech errors that are amenable to therapy. Chapter 5 offers a guide for referring a patient to a cleft palate team. Each chapter begins with a list of key terms relevant to the material presented.

Linda D. Vallino
Dennis M. Ruscello
David J. Zajac

■ Acknowledgments

I would like to express my gratitude to the many people who saw me through this book. These wonderful people provided support and encouragement, talked things over, read (and reread) drafts, offered comments and great suggestions, and made me laugh.

To Denny and David, you are the best! I cherish our longtime and unconditional friendship, and admire your scholarly contributions in the area of cleft palate—I always learn something from you.

I would like to thank the children and their families and the young adults who graciously agreed to be a part of this text. All of them told me that if they can help students and new SLPs learn about cleft palate, then they wanted to have a part in it! And they did. Thank you Cindy Brodoway and Brad Gelman for masterfully videorecording many of the sessions. Cindy, the cover of this book is filled with your fantastic photographs of some very special people. I am most appreciative of your time and talent.

Thanks to Kalie Koscielak and everyone else at Plural Publishing for supporting this idea and for your patience throughout the process, and to all the reviewers who took the time to review the draft of this *Resource*. Your thoughtful comments were positive, constructive, and beneficial.

Last, I am able to do what I truly enjoy because of the love and support of my family. Nicholas, Caroline, John, and Eleanor are four extraordinary children who have grown up to be four extraordinary adults. Then there is my adoring husband, Joe, who is always at the heart of my adventures. You're awesome!

Linda D. Vallino
Wilmington,
Delaware

■ Reviewers

Plural Publishing, Inc. and the authors would like to thank the following reviewers for taking the time to provide their valuable feedback during the development process:

Anne Bedwinek, PhD, CCC-SLP
Adjunct Associate Professor
Department of Communication
  Science & Disorders
The University of Missouri
Columbia, Missouri

Kate Bunton, PhD, CCC-SLP
Associate Professor
Speech, Language, and Hearing
  Sciences
University of Arizona
Tucson, Arizona

Dana R. Collins, PhD, CCC-SLP
Associate Professor
Department of Communication
  Sciences and Disorders
University of Minnesota Duluth
Duluth, Minnesota

John Wm. Folkins, PhD
Professor
Department of Communication
  Sciences and Disorders
Bowling Green State University
Bowling Green, Ohio

Nancy Gauvin, EdD, CCC-SLP
Clinical Assistant Professor

Department of Communication
  Sciences and Disorders
University of Vermont
Burlington, Vermont

**Jennifer M. Glassman, PhD,
CCC-SLP, CHES**
Assistant Professor
Speech-Language Pathology
University of Toledo
Toledo, Ohio

Carol L. Koch, EdD, CCC-SLP
Associate Professor
Communication Sciences and
  Disorders
Samford University
Birmingham, Alabama

Brenda Louw, DPhil, SLP
Professor and Chair
Department Audiology and Speech-
  Language Pathology
East Tennessee State University
Johnson City, Tennessee

Jayanti Ray, PhD, CCC-SLP
Professor
Communication Disorders
Southeast Missouri State University
Cape Girardeau, Missouri

Gale B. Rice, PhD, CCC-SLP
Dean, College of Education and
   Allied Health Professions
Fontbonne University
Speech-Language Pathologist,
   Craniofacial Anomalies Team
The University of Missouri
Columbia, Missouri

Jeff Searl, PhD, CCC-SLP
Associate Professor

Department of Communicative
   Sciences and Disorders
Michigan State University
East Lansing, Michigan

**Natalie R. Wombacher, MS,
CCC-SLP**
Speech-Language Pathologist
Craniofacial Anomalies Program
University of Michigan
Ann Arbor, Michigan

List of Abbreviations

ACPA	American Cleft Palate-Craniofacial Association
ANE	Audible nasal emission
ANF	Anterior nasal fricative
ASHA	American Speech-Language-Hearing Association
CLP	Cleft lip and palate
EMT	Enhanced Milieu Training
EMT/PE	Enhanced Milieu Training with Phonological Emphasis
ENT	Ear, Nose, and Throat
HIPAA	Health Insurance Portability Accountability Act
KR	Knowledge of Results
MADO	Maxillary advancement using distraction osteogenesis
NA	None apparent
NE	Nasal emission
NF1	Neurofibromatosis, type 1
NSOME	Nonspeech oral motor exercises
NT	Nasal turbulence
OME	Otitis media with effusion
OSA	Obstructive sleep apnea
PE	Pressure-equalization
PNF	Posterior nasal fricative
PSNE	Phoneme-specific nasal emission
SLP	Speech-language pathologist
SNHL	Sensorineural hearing loss

T&A	Tonsillectomy & adenoidectomy
VP	Velopharyngeal
VPD	Velopharyngeal dysfunction
VPI	Velopharyngeal inadequacy
WFL	Within functional limits
WNL	Within normal limits

■ Legend to Audio and Video Samples

Chapter 3
Section 1
Speech Features Commonly Associated With Cleft Palate and Velopharyngeal Dysfunction

Resonance
Audio 3.1.1   Normal nasal resonance
Audio 3.1.2   Slight hypernasality but within functional limits
Audio 3.1.3   Mild hypernasality
Audio 3.1.4   Mild-moderate hypernasality
Audio 3.1.5   Moderate hypernasality
Audio 3.1.6   Moderate hypernasality, oral distortions
Audio 3.1.7   Severe hypernasality
Audio 3.1.8   Mild hyponasality
Audio 3.1.9   Mild-moderate hyponasality
Audio 3.1.10 Mixed hyper-hyponasality

Nasal Air Emission
Audio 3.1.11 Audible nasal air emission (ANE)
Audio 3.1.12 ANE on /s/ and /z/ segments
Audio 3.1.13 ANE
Audio 3.1.14 ANE
Audio 3.1.15 Nasal turbulence

Articulation Errors Within the Oral Cavity
Obligatory (Adaptive) Oral Distortions
Audio 3.1.16 Anterior sibilant and affricate distortions
Audio 3.1.17 Interdental /s/
Audio 3.1.18 Interdental /s/
Audio 3.1.19 Fronting on fricatives and affricates
Audio 3.1.20 Dentalized /s/
Audio 3.1.21 Lateral /s/ distortions
Audio 3.1.22 Palatalized stop during production of /t/ (Note: We acknowledge that others have considered this as a compensatory misarticulation, and as discussed in the text it is best characterized in some cases as an obligatory oral distortion.
Audio 3.1.23 Dentalized alveolar and palatal sounds

Articulation Errors Outside the Oral Cavity
Compensatory (Maladaptive) Articulation

Other Unusual Articulations

Phonatory Disorders

Section 2
Audio Case Studies: Guided Practice

Audio 3.2.6   9-year old female with hypernasality following tonsillectomy and adenoidectomy

Audio 3.2.7   15-year-old male with Pierre Robin sequence and repaired cleft palate with hypernasality, and generalized backing of alveolar sounds

Audio 3.2.8   7-year-old female with repaired left unilateral cleft lip and bifid uvula and posterior nasal turbulence

Audio 3.2.9   15-year-old female with left unilateral cleft lip and palate with moderate hypernasality, audible nasal emission, and anterior nasal frication on sibilants

Audio 3.2.10   9-year-old boy with right hemifacial macrosomia with posterior nasal fricatives

Audio 3.2.11   8-year-old female with submucous cleft palate with mild hypernasality, audible nasal air emission, interdentalized sibilants, an unusual gr/w substitution.

Audio 3.2.12   8-year-old female who underwent surgery for oral tumor that included removal of portions of the soft and hard palate that were repaired. She has very mild hypernasal speech and normal articulation with hard glottal attacks on counting from 80 to 90.

Audio 3.2.13   13-year-old female with a profound, rising to mild mixed hearing loss with moderate hypernasality

Audio 3.2.14   19-year-old female with muscular dystrophy and flaccid dysarthria with moderate hypernasality, and imprecise articulation

Audio 3.2.15   12-year-old female without a visible cleft lip or palate with hypernasal speech following tonsillectomy and adenoidectomy

Audio 3.2.16   6-year-old male with repaired right unilateral cleft lip and palate with moderate hypernasality, audible nasal air emission, and reduced loudness. He also produced /s/ on inspiration.

Audio 3.2.17   14-year-old male with repaired bilateral cleft lip and palate with moderate hypernasality, audible nasal air emission, weak pressure consonants, and oral distortions

Audio 3.2.18   6-year-old male with a complete cleft palate with moderate hypernasality and compensatory articulation errors

Audio 3.2.19   3.5-year-old male with repaired left unilateral cleft lip and palate with mild hypernasality, audible nasal air emission, high pitch, and developmental errors

Audio 3.2.20   4-year-old male with repaired left unilateral cleft lip and palate with moderate hypernasality, audible nasal air emission, and stopping errors

Section 3
Audio Case Studies: Independent Practice

Audio 3.3.1   20-year-old male with repaired bilateral cleft lip and palate with normal resonance

Audio 3.3.2   12-year-old male with repaired left cleft lip and palate with slight hyponasality and lateral distortions

Audio 3.3.3   7-year-old male with repaired bilateral cleft lip and palate with mild to moderate hypernasality, and lateralization of the alveolar and palatal fricatives and affricates

Audio 3.3.4   9-year-old male with Stickler syndrome with mild to moderate hypernasality

Audio 3.3.5   11-year-old female with 22q11.2 deletion syndrome with mild hypernasality, mild hoarseness, and speech sound errors

Audio 3.3.6   11-year-old male with a repaired left unilateral cleft lip and palate with mild hypernasality, intermittent audible nasal air emission, and normal articulation

Audio 3.3.7   4-year-old female without cleft palate with posterior nasal fricatives characterized by nasal turbulence for affricates.

Audio 3.3.8   15-year-old male with popliteal pterygium syndrome and repaired cleft palate with moderate hypernasality, audible nasal air emission, glottal stops, and palatal fricatives and affricates

Audio 3.3.9   17-year-old female with repaired right unilateral cleft lip and palate after maxillary advancement. She has mild hypernasality and intermittent audible nasal air emission.

Audio 3.3.10   6-year-old with repaired bilateral cleft lip and palate with moderate hypernasality, intermittent audible nasal air emission, and compensatory articulation errors

Audio 3.3.11   18-year-old young adult with repaired left unilateral cleft lip and palate withmoderate hypernasality, audible nasal air emission, and weak pressure consonants

Audio 3.3.12   8-year-old female with Stickler syndrome and repaired isolated cleft palate with moderate hypernaslity and audible turbulence

Audio 3.3.13   13-year-old male with Klippel-Feil syndrome and repaired left unilateral cleft lip and palate with hyponasality, fronting of alveolar and palatal sounds, and other articulation errors

Audio 3.3.14   7-year-old male with repaired bilateral cleft lip and palate with moderate hypernasality and lateralization of sibilants

Audio 3.3.15   7-year-old female with neurofibromatosis with severe hypernasality, imprecise articulation, and pitch variations

Audio 3.3.16   Almost 4-year-old male with repaired left unilateral cleft
                lip and palate withmoderate hypernasality, nasal fricatives,
                glottal stops, sound deletions, and severe hoarseness
Audio 3.3.17   6-year-old female with submucous cleft palate with
                moderate hypernasality, nasal fricative, /r/ distortion, and
                mild hoarseness
Audio 3.3.18   3-year-old male with repaired right unilateral cleft lip
                and palate with moderate hypernasality, audible nasal
                air emission, compensatory articulation errors, and
                developmental speech errors
Audio 3.3.19   9-year-old male with repaired right unilateral cleft lip
                and palate with moderate hypernasality, compensatory
                articulation errors including glottal stops, pharyngeal
                fricatives, and pharyngeal affricates
Audio 3.3.20   This is the same patient presented in Audio 3.3.19 one year
                after push-back revision palatoplasty with buccal flaps to
                improve VPD. He has normal resonance and persistent
                compensatory errors.

Section 4
Video Case Studies: Independent Practice

Video 3.4.1   2-year-old female with isolated cleft palate with normal
               resonance and age-appropriate articulation development.
Video 3.4.2   6-year-old male with isolated cleft palate with essentially
               normal resonance albeit a slight hint of hyponasality on
               nasal consonants, and developmental articulation errors
               unrelated to cleft palate.
Video 3.4.3   14-year-old female with left unilateral cleft lip and palate
               with resonance that is within functional limits during
               citation but demonstrates an increase in hypernasality
               during conversational speech. Her videonasoendoscopic
               assessment is also shown.
Video 3.4.4   6-year-old male with right unilateral cleft lip and palate
               with mild hypernasality, facial grimace, and oral distortions.
Video 3.4.5   11-year-old male with bilateral cleft lip and palate with mild
               hypernasal speech, audible nasal air emission, nasal grimace,
               obligatory oral distortions, and hoarse voice quality.
Video 3.4.6   18-year-old female with left unilateral cleft lip and palate with
               moderate hypernasal speech, audible nasal air emission, and
               nasal grimace. She is shown again after surgery to improve
               speech and resonance.
Video 3.4.7   11-year-old male without cleft palate with mild-moderate
               hypernasality, and nasal turbulence.

We dedicate this publication to our families who have always supported us in our academic and clinical endeavors. In addition, we acknowledge and dedicate this work to Drs. Betty Jane McWilliams, Betty Jane Philips, and Ralph Shelton, who are pioneers in cleft care and whose work inspired us to embark upon this project. Finally, this is dedicated to all of those who were born with a cleft condition and benefited from the services of cleft palate–craniofacial teams and different community care specialists.

1

Resonance and Speech Problems

- Nasal Substitutions
- Nasalized Plosives
- Obligatory (Adaptive) Oral Distortions
- Otitis Media With Effusion (OME)
- Palatalized Tongue-Tip Stops/Fricatives (Mid-Dorsum Palatal)
- Pharyngeal Affricates
- Pharyngeal Fricatives
- Pharyngeal Stops
- Phoneme-Specific Nasal Emission (PSNE)
- Resonance
- Velarized Nasals/Liquids
- Velopharyngeal Dysfunction (VPD)
- Velopharyngeal Inadequacy (VPI)
- Velopharyngeal Incompetency
- Velopharyngeal Insufficiency
- Weak Pressure Consonants

■ Introduction

There are three ways that the speech-language pathologist (SLP) studies speech production, and these are physiologic, acoustic, and perceptual (see Chapter 2). Each study method is important in understanding normal and disordered speech production, because of the different information that each provides. However, the decisive test for a person with a communication disorder(s) is the perceptual impact of the problem. What is the impression of a person with a communication disorder that other speakers form when engaging with them in verbal communication? This is particularly important for speakers with cleft palate because they may present with problems that affect different speech production subsystems. Thus, the ear is the most important clinical tool for the SLP who must develop a perceptual frame of reference for the different speech disorders that may be present in a speaker with cleft palate. That is, one must listen and be able to identify the feature(s) of the communication disorder in a reliable manner and formulate appropriate diagnostic and treatment plans. We must note, however, that some speech characteristics associated with cleft palate are difficult to reliably identify with the ear alone. Palatalized stops (or mid-dorsum palatal stops), for example, are quite difficult even for experienced SLPs to identify (Santelmann, Sussman, & Chapman, 1999). Likewise, although most can easily recognize the distinctive sound of a learned nasal fricative, a similar or even identical sound can occur as an obligatory consequence of velopharyngeal dysfunction (VPD). In these cases, the use of objective instrumentation is essential to make appropriate diagnostic and management plans. We provide examples in Chapter 3 to illustrate the use of acoustic analysis to confirm perceptual identification of nasal fricatives.

We begin this chapter with an overview of the velopharyngeal valving mechanism for speech. This is followed by a description of the types of speech problems associated with cleft palate and other problems of VPD, including resonance, nasal air emission, articulation, and phonation. Other important considerations, including hearing problems and other potential coexisting speech problems unrelated to the cleft, will be discussed.

■ A Note on Terminology

In describing problems of velopharyngeal closure, there is often confusion about terminology usage. Throughout this *Resource*, the term *velopharyngeal dysfunction* (VPD) is used to refer to a problem of velopharyngeal closure. *Velopharyngeal inadequacy* (VPI) is a synonymous term that also denotes abnormal velopharyngeal function (Folkins, 1988). It is important to emphasize that both terms are generic and that neither one specifies a cause of the problem.

There are, however, terms used to describe impaired velopharyngeal function based on anatomical or physiologic referents. *Velopharyngeal insufficiency* (anatomic) is used to denote impaired velopharyngeal function that occurs as a result of insufficient tissue to accomplish velopharyngeal closure. *Velopharyngeal incompetence* (physiologic) denotes a neurologic etiology that results in impaired motor control of the velopharyngeal mechanism.

Because we are relying on perceptual judgments about the adequacy of speech and not using instrumentation to identify the structural or neurological processes causing impaired velopharyngeal function (Folkins, 1988), the term *VPD* used in this text to refer to problems of velopharyngeal closure is appropriate.

■ Overview of the Velopharyngeal Mechanism

The complexity of the velopharyngeal (VP) mechanism is well recognized and appreciated, the details of which are beyond the scope of this *Resource*. The aim of this section is to provide the SLP with an overview of the of the VP mechanism during the production of speech. For the interested reader, comprehensive descriptions of VP anatomy and function can be found in texts such as Zemlin (1998); Peterson-Falzone, Hardin-Jones, and Karnell (2010); and Zajac and Vallino (2017).

Anatomy

The palate is made up of the hard palate anteriorly and the soft palate posteriorly (Figure 1–1). The hard palate is the bony structure that forms the roof of the mouth and floor of the nasal cavity. The soft palate or velum extends beyond the hard palate and is continuous with the uvula, the pedunculated structure at the end of the velum.

The velopharyngeal mechanism is composed of the velum, lateral pharyngeal walls, and the posterior pharyngeal wall (back wall of the throat). The space surrounded by these structures is referred to as the velopharyngeal port (Figure 1–2).

There are five muscle pairs of the velum and pharynx that are involved in velopharyngeal movement. They are the

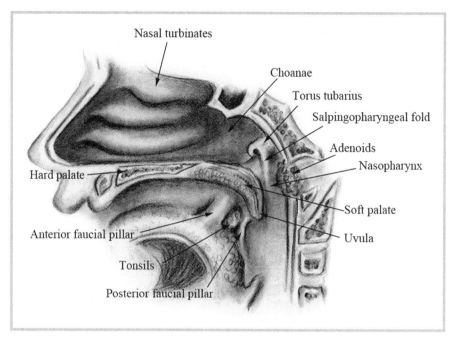

Figure 1–1. Lateral view of the oral and nasal cavities and nasopharynx. *Source*: Reprinted with permission from Zajac, D. J., and Vallino, L. D. (2017). *Evaluation and management of cleft lip and palate.* San Diego, CA: Plural Publishing.

levator veli palatini, palatoglossus, musculus uvulus, palato-pharyngeus, and tensor veli palatini (Figure 1–3).

The *levator veli palatini* is the primary muscle respon-sible for elevating and retracting the velum. The *palatoglos-sus* muscle is antagonistic to the levator muscle, and when contracted, it lowers the velum during speech and also acts to elevate the tongue during bolus preparation and transport. The *musculus uvulus* adds bulk to the velum and may stiffen to provide firm contact to the posterior pharyngeal wall. The horizontal fibers of the *palatopharyngeus* muscle provide sphincter action to orient the lateral pharyngeal walls medi-ally, and its vertical fibers may lower the velum and elevate the pharynx/larynx during deglutition. The muscle responsible for medial displacement of the lateral pharyngeal walls is the

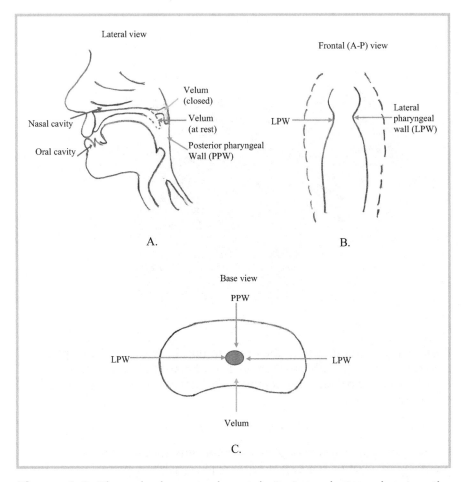

Figure 1–2. The velopharyngeal portal. **A.** Lateral view showing the velum and posterior pharyngeal wall. **B.** Frontal or anteroposterior (A-P) view showing the lateral pharyngeal walls. **C.** Base view showing the entire velopharyngeal portal. The circle is illustrative of the velopharyngeal portal.

superior constrictor. The *tensor veli palatini* muscle is also often included as a muscle involved in velopharyngeal movement. However, the primary purpose of this muscle is to open or dilate the eustachian tubes (Dickson & Maue-Dickson, 1982; Rood & Doyle, 1978).

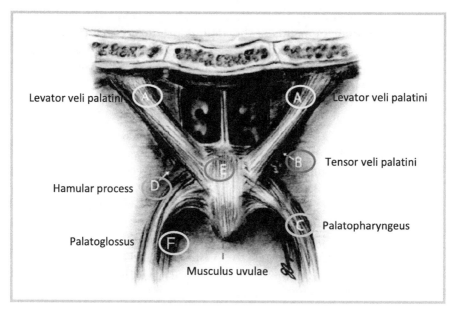

Levator veli palatini

Levator veli palatini

Tensor veli palatini

Hamular process

Palatopharyngeus

Palatoglossus

Musculus uvulae

Figure 1–3. Posterior view of the muscles of the velum and pharynx. *Source:* Reprinted with permission from Zajac, D. J., and Vallino, L. D. (2017). *Evaluation and management of cleft lip and palate.* San Diego, CA: Plural Publishing.

Function

The velopharyngeal mechanism functions as an aerodynamic-acoustic valve that serves to create a tight seal between the velum and posterior pharyngeal wall in order to separate the oral and nasal cavities (Zajac & Vallino, 2017). At rest, when the mouth is closed and during nasal breathing, the velum may rest against the base of the tongue. Velopharyngeal closure is a complex coordinated process that is necessary in order for a speaker to produce speech in a correct manner. It is dependent upon the system's capacity to couple and decouple the nasal cavity from the oral cavity (Peterson-Falzone et al., 2010; Zemlin, 1998). In English, there are three nasal sounds /m, n, ŋ/ that require oral-nasal coupling (i.e., an open velopharyngeal port), while the oral speech sounds require oral-nasal decoupling (i.e., separation of the oral and nasal cavities). This coupling and decoupling of the nasal and oral cavities is referred to as velopharyngeal valving, and it continuously adjusts to the phonetic demands of the sounds produced (Peterson-Falzone et al., 2010). Figures 1–4A and 1–4B show the velopharyngeal valve at rest during quiet breathing and during complete velopharyngeal closure during speech.

Velopharyngeal closure is frequently characterized as a sphincteric action (Skolnick, McCall, & Barnes, 1973) (see Figure 1–2). As noted earlier, the primary mechanism for velopharyngeal closure is accomplished by elevation and retraction of the velum. Movement of the pharyngeal walls contributes to the sphincteric activity involved in velopharyngeal closure (Skolnick et al., 1973). The lateral pharyngeal walls move medially (inwardly) to abut against the edges of the velum and the posterior pharyngeal wall moves anteriorly. The relative contributions of the velum, lateral pharyngeal walls, and the posterior pharyngeal wall vary from person to person, thus resulting in different patterns of closure for speech. Complete VP closure allows for the buildup of air pressure within the oral cavity that is obstructed or nearly obstructed by the lips, tongue, and teeth that is subsequently released to produce oral pressure consonants such as plosives, fricatives, and affricates.

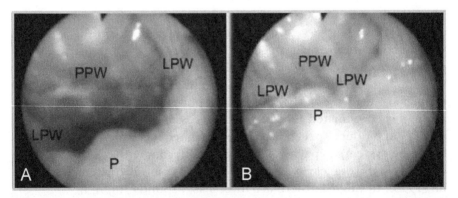

Figure 1–4. Velopharyngeal valve as seen by flexible nasopharyngoscopy (1) open during rest and (2) closed during articulation. P = palate; LPW = lateral pharyngeal wall; PPW = posterior pharyngeal wall. *Source:* Reprinted with permission from Abdel-Aziz, M. (2014). Velopharyngeal insufficiency in children. *Austin Journal of Otolaryngology, 1,* 1–4.

Velopharyngeal Dysfunction

Velopharyngeal dysfunction (VPD) occurs as a result of the inability to adequately separate the oral and nasal cavities during the production of oral speech sounds (Figures 1–5A and 1–5B). It is the major etiological cause of resonance and speech sound disorders of speakers with cleft palate (Peterson-Falzone et al., 2010; Zajac & Vallino, 2017).

There are many causes of VPD, all of which will affect speech. The most common cause is cleft palate. VPD can also persist after primary surgical repair of the palate or present in some patients with unrepaired overt or occult submucous cleft palate (Zajac & Vallino, 2017). For others, however, who do not have a cleft palate, VPD may be caused by other structural anomalies of the palate other than a cleft, a neurogenic disorder, or surgery (e.g., adenoidectomy), and in some cases, the etiology is unknown. The multiple causal factors indicate that the population of patients with VPD is quite heterogeneous, and the SLP who works exclusively in a cleft palate clinic will see a diverse group of patients with respect to etiology. That is, not all patients will exhibit overt clefts but any number of different problems. Similarly, practitioners who do not see

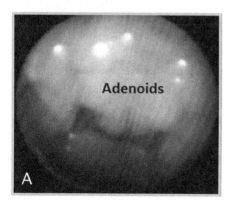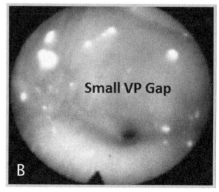

Figure 1–5. Nasoendoscopic image of velopharyngeal dysfunction (VPD). **A.** Open during rest. **B.** Incomplete velopharyngeal closure in a speaker with velopharyngeal dysfunction. *Source:* Reprinted with permission from Zajac, D. J., and Vallino, L. D. (2017). *Evaluation and management of cleft lip and palate.* San Diego, CA: Plural Publishing.

patients with VPD on a frequents basis must be vigilant to the symptoms, since there are a number of different etiological factors responsible for VPD. The etiological factors associated with VPD are shown in Table 1–1.

In some speakers, what might be considered as VPD is actually a problem of articulatory mislearning. These speakers learn to produce certain oral pressure sounds such as sibilants by closing the oral cavity and shunting the air through the nose. Of diagnostic importance, these speakers typically demonstrate adequate VP function on all other oral pressure sounds. To be sure, some of these speakers do not have cleft palate or any known structural problem. This type of error is called a nasal fricative (referred to by some as phoneme-specific nasal emission), which will be described later in this chapter.

■ Communication Problems Associated With Cleft Palate

Some patients with cleft palate will exhibit normal-sounding resonance and articulation after primary cleft palate repair. Others, however, will not have normal-sounding speech. Some patients may present with obligatory symptoms that occur as a direct consequence of VPD (e.g., hypernasal resonance, audible nasal air emission, nasalized plosives). Some patients may present with learned maladaptive articulations that occur as compensation for VPD (e.g., glottal stops, pharyngeal fricatives). The term "maladaptive" refers to gross changes in place of articulation that severely affects intelligibility (see Figure 1–6). Some patients may present with obligatory articulations that occur as a direct consequence of oral structural anomalies (e.g., interdental or lateral distortions). These types of articulation are sometimes referred to as "adaptive" because the speaker does not attempt to compensate for the structural anomaly by changing place of articulation (Peterson-Falzone, Trost-Cardamone, Harding-Jones, & Karnell, 2001). Still others may demonstrate problems that are unrelated to the cleft such as mislearned articulatory productions, phonological errors, and

Table 1–1. Etiological Factors Associated With Velopharyngeal Dysfunction (VPD)

Structural	Neurogenic	Surgically Induced	Other Causes
Overt unrepaired cleft palate	Dysarthria	Failure to achieve velopharyngeal closure after primary palate repair	Postradiation fibrosis
Submucous cleft palate	Apraxia	Failure to achieve velopharyngeal closure after pharyngoplasty	Pharmacological induction of VPD
Occult submucous cleft palate	Hypotonia	Maxillary advancement	Post-tonsillectomy cauterization
Capacious (deep) pharynx	Stroke	Adenoidectomy	Idiopathic (unknown origin)
Short velum	Cranial nerve IX, X, XI damage	Maxillary resection (i.e., ablative surgery)	Sensorineural hearing loss
Velar hypoplasia	Velar fatigue		
Adenoid involution	Progressive neurological disorders (i.e., amyotrophic lateral sclerosis [ALS])		
Irregular adenoid pad			
Excessively large tonsils interfering with lateral pharyngeal wall movement			

continues

Table 1–1. *continued*

Structural	Neurogenic	Surgically Induced	Other Causes
Posterior pillar webbing			
Tumors of the oral cavity and/ or nasopharynx			
Palatal trauma			

motor speech disorders. Any finally, it is not unusual for a speaker with VPD to exhibit a phonatory disorder.

The potential for numerous types of problems that may affect resonance, nasal air emission, and articulation, requires that the SLP have the necessary background knowledge and auditory perceptual skills to understand and identify the different disorders associated with VPD. In the ensuing sections, we will describe the speech problems occurring as a direct result of VPD and other maladaptive patterns of speech. Other potential coexisting speech problems unrelated to the cleft condition will also be discussed.

Resonance Characteristics

Resonance is a complex acoustic-perceptual phenomenon (Zajac & Vallino, 2017). In humans, resonance occurs when a vibrating sound source (vocal folds) excites an air-filled cavity such as the pharynx, oral cavity, and nasal cavity. Resonance is determined by the frequency of vocal fold vibration and the characteristics of the resonating cavities. Because voicing is required, resonance only occurs on voiced consonants and vowels, not voiceless consonants. For speakers without structural anomalies and adequate velopharyngeal closure, resonance during the production of vowels and voiced oral consonants occurs primarily in the pharyngeal and oral cavities (Zajac & Vallino, 2017). During the production of nasal consonants and nasalized vowels when the velum is lowered, the nasal cavity becomes an additional resonator (Zajac & Vallino, 2017).

There are four types of resonance disorders that an individual with cleft palate can exhibit: hypernasality, hyponasality, mixed hyper-hyponasality, and cul-de-sac.

Hypernasality

Hypernasality is the most defining speech feature of patients with cleft palate who have VPD (Zajac & Vallino, 2017). It is characterized by excessive nasal resonance that occurs as a result of inappropriate coupling between the oral and nasal cavities during the production of vowels and vocalic consonants. SLPs less experienced with resonance disorders often confuse hypernasality with nasal air emission. Readers should be mindful that hypernasality is a resonance disorder and nasal air emission is strictly an airflow disorder that may occur with or without hypernasality. This is detailed in the section on nasal air emission, which appears later in this chapter.

Hyponasality

Hyponasality is the reduction of nasal resonance that is perceived during the production of the nasal speech sounds /m/, /n/, and /ŋ/. It is generally caused by an incomplete blockage of the nasal passages, or partial occlusion at the posterior entrance to the nasal passages. It is tempting at times for the SLP to believe that the patient presenting with hyponasality must have an adequate velopharyngeal mechanism when, in fact, he or she may have VPD. In these cases, the effects of VPD may be obscured by the presence of conditions causing hyponasal speech (e.g., enlarged adenoid pad, large nasal turbinates, nasal polyps, shallow nasopharynx, choanal atresia, wide pharyngeal flap) (McWilliams, Shelton, & Morris, 1990). Where cases such as these exist, the perceptual effects of VPD on speech become evident once the condition causing the hyponasality is corrected.

Hyper-Hyponasality (Mixed Resonance)

It is possible that some individuals with cleft palate exhibit both hyper- and hyponasality. The hypernasal speech results from VPD and the hyponasality from some type of nasal obstruction that allows partial nasal coupling, but it is not sufficient to maintain normal nasal speech sound production.

Cul-de-Sac

The final resonance category is that of cul-de-sac resonance. It is a lack of normal oral resonance that often results in a muffled, nasopharyngeal quality (Zajac & Vallino, 2017). Kummer (2014) calls this pharyngeal cul-de-sac and attributes the quality to enlarged tonsils that impede efficient oral resonance. Some patients with syndromes such as Treacher Collins may exhibit this quality due to a small and retracted mandible (Vallino, Peterson-Falzone, & Napoli, 2006). Still others consider cul-de-sac a variant of hyponasal resonance caused by anterior obstruction of the nasal cavity (Peterson-Falzone et al., 2001). Peterson-Falzone et al. (2001) remarked that this type of cul-de-sac resonance can be simulated by first producing "mi" normally and then with the nostrils occluded. There is, however, little consensus regarding these two clinical cul-de-sac terms and little objective-perceptual research on this type of resonance (Zajac & Vallino, 2017). In this *Resource*, we use the term *cul-de-sac* to refer to a lack of normal oral resonance.

 Audio samples 3.1.1 through 3.1.10 in the Resonance module are from speakers who exhibit normal resonance and various types and severity of resonance imbalance.

Nasal Air Emission

Nasal air emission is the second most defining speech feature of patients with cleft palate and VPD (Zajac & Vallino, 2017). Nasal air emission—similar to articulation errors described later in this chapter—can be either obligatory (passive) or learned (active). It must be emphasized that nasal air emission due to obligatory and learned causes can sound similar or even identical, and both can occur in a given speaker. It is for these reasons that there have been a variety of terms, often confusing and/or inaccurate, used to describe nasal air emission. In this section, we describe nasal air emission that results from VPD as an obligatory speech symptom. We describe nasal air emission that results from learned misarticulations later in this chapter.

Obligatory nasal emission is defined as the unwanted passage of air into the nasal cavity during the production of high-pressure oral consonants—plosives, fricatives, and affricates—as a function of VPD or an oronasal fistula. It presents as bursts of nasal airflow or continuous nasal airflow during production of stops and continuant consonants, respectively. Whereas hypernasality is a resonance phenomenon that occurs on vowels and voiced consonants, nasal air emission is an aerodynamic event that occurs exclusively on pressure obstruent consonants, especially voiceless consonants (Zajac & Vallino, 2017). Although the presence of nasal emission is evidence of VPD, nasal emission is *not* synonymous with hypernasality. Hypernasality is actually associated with little nasal airflow due to resistance caused by the vibrating vocal folds. Even though these two conditions can co-occur in a speaker, these are distinct perceptual symptoms that occur on different speech segments for different physiologic reasons (Zajac & Vallino, 2017) (Table 1–2).

Obligatory nasal air emission can occur across a continuum from visible only (not perceptually audible) to audible to turbulent. In the absence of neuromotor dysfunction, oronasal fistula, or articulatory mislearning (see section on articulation), nasal emission is a direct consequence of VPD (Zajac & Vallino, 2017). When present, it can be seen as fogging or misting on a mirror when placed under the nose during high-pressure consonant production.

Many SLPs have accepted the terms *audible* and *turbulent* to describe two distinct forms of audible nasal air emission. Audible nasal air emission is usually associated with relatively large VP gaps. In this situation, airflow becomes turbulent and causes frication-like noise as it passes through the anterior nasal valve, the smallest cross-sectional area of the nose (Proctor, 1982). The sound of audible nasal air emission can

Table 1–2. Distinguishing Characteristics of Hypernasality and Nasal Air Emission

Hypernasality	*Nasal Air Emission*
Resonance phenomenon	Aerodynamic phenomenon
Occurs on vowels and voiced consonants	Occurs on obstruent consonants, especially voiceless consonants
Associated with little nasal airflow	Nasal emission (NE) can be visible only, audible, or turbulent • Visual NE—detected by mirror • Audible NE—turbulence created at anterior nasal valve • Turbulent NE—turbulence created at VP port (often with tissue flutter)

Source: Reprinted with permission from Zajac, D. J., and Vallino, L. D. (2017). *Evaluation and management of cleft lip and palate.* San Diego, CA: Plural Publishing.

be simulated by forcefully exhaling through the nose. Nasal turbulence is usually associated with a relatively small VP gap. In this situation, airflow becomes turbulent and causes relatively louder frication-like noise as it passes through a small VP valve. Peterson-Falzone, Hardin-Jones, and Karnell (2001) have importantly noted that extra noises often accompany nasal turbulence. These extra noises may arise from displacement of mucous in the VP port and/or vibration (flutter) of velar tissue. Kummer (2014) referred to nasal turbulence as "nasal rustle" and attributed its distinctive sound to the bubbling of secretions in a small velopharyngeal port. A study by Zajac and Preisser (2016), however, presented acoustic-spectral evidence showing that quasi-periodic flutter was the major perceptual component of obligatory nasal turbulence. This flutter resembles a raspberry-like noise. Zajac and Preisser suggested that flutter was due to tissue vibration as suggested by Peterson-Falzone et al. (2001).

A nasal grimace may be observed in some patients with severe VPD and audible nasal air emission. McWilliams and

Cohn (2002) state that a nasal grimace may occur as a compensatory response to prevent the obligatory loss of air through the nose. Warren (1986) hypothesized that it may occur in an attempt to maintain oral air pressure at adequate levels for consonant production. It is typically characterized by constriction of the nares during production of high-pressure oral segments in response to obligatory nasal air emission. In addition, we have observed one young child with repaired bilateral cleft lip and palate who appeared to grimace more severely during speech segments that required either lip protrusion or spreading. In this case, the grimace may have occurred secondarily as a result of biomechanical linkage of the lip and nose.

Some speakers with severe VPD and audible nasal air emission may also exhibit weak and nasalized plosives. There is an attempt to impound air orally, but the VPD, if severe, prevents the development of adequate intraoral pressure because air is lost through the nose. In severe cases, production of a plosive such as /b/ may almost sound like /m/. Similarly, production of /d/ may sound like /n/. Occlusion of the nostrils in such cases generally results in adequate intraoral pressure buildup and perceptually adequate production of oral pressure sounds. As discussed later in this chapter, extreme nasalization of /b/ and /d/ due to weak oral pressure should not be confused with true nasal substitutions (e.g., m/b) due to a phonological disorder.

When discussing weak pressure consonants, a cautionary point needs to be made. That is, weak or reduced intraoral pressure cannot actually be heard, making it difficult to perceptually qualify. What seems to actually be perceived are reduced intensity of stop release bursts and reduced intensity of fricative noise. This is perhaps most evident when there is severe hypernasality and reduced loudness. Clinically, suspected weak or reduced oral pressure consonants should be confirmed by an instrumental technique such as pressure-flow. Unfortunately, few SLPs have access to this equipment in their clinic.

Audio samples 3.1.11 through 3.1.15 in the Nasal Emission module are from speakers who exhibit audible nasal air emission and/or nasal turbulence.

■ Articulation

When discussing the articulation problems of patients with clefts, we need to distinguish the classificatory terms *obligatory (adaptive)* and *compensatory (maladaptive)*. The etiology, place of articulation, and characteristics are very different from each other. In addition, there are some articulation errors such as palatalized stops and nasal fricatives that cannot be easily classified and are discussed later. This can be confusing for students and SLPs less familiar with cleft palate speech. The differential diagnosis between obligatory (adaptive) and compensatory (maladaptive) articulation errors, however, is an important one to make in that recommendations regarding appropriate treatment (i.e., surgery vs. speech therapy) will differ. Therefore, in an attempt to provide a clearer understanding of the various articulation errors that can occur in patients with cleft palate, we first describe errors as occurring either within or outside of the oral cavity and secondarily discuss likely etiology of the errors. As seen in Figure 1–6, we begin with discussion of errors occurring *within* the oral cavity. These include obligatory oral distortions (adaptive errors), backed placement of alveolar sounds, and other uncommon errors such as fricatives produced on inspiration and clicks that accompany and/or replace stops. We then discuss errors occurring *outside* of the oral cavity. These errors tend to affect intelligibility and acceptability more and include the traditional maladaptive compensatory errors produced in the pharynx and glottis and other unusual errors such as nasal fricatives.

Articulation Errors Within the Oral Cavity

Obligatory (Adaptive) Oral Distortions

Dental anomalies and occlusal defects are common in patients with cleft lip and palate (CLP), placing them at risk for oral distortions (Peterson-Falzone et al., 2010; Witzel & Vallino, 1992; Zajac & Vallino, 2017). These particular speech errors are classified as obligatory and adaptive because they unavoidably

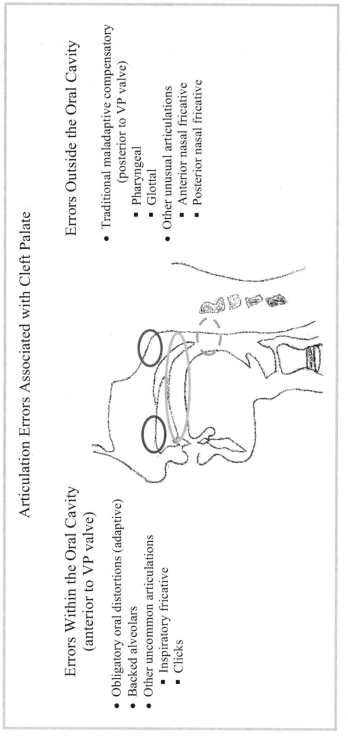

Articulation Errors Associated with Cleft Palate

Errors Within the Oral Cavity (anterior to VP valve)

- Obligatory oral distortions (adaptive)
- Backed alveolars
- Other uncommon articulations
  - Inspiratory fricative
  - Clicks

Errors Outside the Oral Cavity

- Traditional maladaptive compensatory (posterior to VP valve)
  - Pharyngeal
  - Glottal
- Other unusual articulations
  - Anterior nasal fricative
  - Posterior nasal fricative

Figure 1–6. Schematic illustrating the differential articulatory placement of errors produced within the oral cavity (anterior to the VP valve) and errors produced outside the oral cavity.

occur as a consequence of the oral structural defects and the speaker does not attempt to compensate. The sounds most commonly affected by dental and occlusal anomalies are the sibilants /s, z, ʃ, ʒ/ and the affricates /tʃ, dʒ/. In some cases, the tongue-tip alveolar stops /t, d/, nasal /n/, and liquid /l/ may be affected. If the dental/occlusal defect is severe enough to prevent the lips and/or teeth from coming together, then /p, b, m, f, v/ can be produced abnormally.

Dental anomalies are common among patients with CLP, typically occurring on the side of the cleft. The most common anomalies are congenitally missing maxillary lateral incisors and supernumerary or extra teeth. Patients with these dental conditions can have difficulty with the accurate production of /s/ and /z/. It is also not unusual to find variations in tooth size, shape, number, structure and formation, location (ectopic), and eruption timing (Tortora, Meazzini, Garattini, & Brusati, 2008).

There is substantial evidence to show that dental and occlusal defects can distort articulation. Occlusion can be classified as dental or skeletal. Dental occlusion refers to the natural fitting together of the upper and lower teeth when the jaws are closed. Angle classified occlusions using the relationship between the maxillary and mandibular first molars. In a normal dental occlusion (Class I occlusion), the mesiobuccal cusp of the maxillary first molar rests in the buccal groove of the mandibular first molar when the jaws are closed (Figure 1–7A). A deviation from the normal relationship is considered a malocclusion. In a Class II malocclusion the upper molar is anterior to the lower molar (Figure 1–7B) and in a Class III malocclusion the upper molar is posterior to the lower molar (Figure 1–7C) (Zajac & Vallino, 2017).

An open bite occurs when the maxillary and mandibular incisors do not make contact. This typically causes the tongue to protrude through the opening between the teeth, which results in the fronting of the alveolars and possibly palatals (Zajac & Vallino, 2017). An open-bite malocclusion is shown in Figure 1–8.

Skeletal malocclusion refers to the incorrect relationship between the upper and lower jaws. That is, they are not in appropriate alignment (Zajac & Vallino, 2017). Skeletal rela-

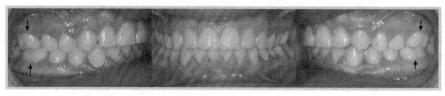

A

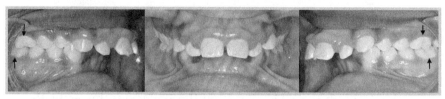

B

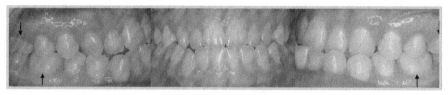

C

Figure 1–7. **A.** Angle Class I occlusion. **B.** Angle Class II malocclusion. **C.** Angle Class III malocclusion. *Source:* Courtesy of the Department of Orthodontics, University of North Carolina at Chapel Hill. Reprinted with permission from Zajac, D. J., and Vallino, L. D. (2017). *Evaluation and management of cleft lip and palate.* San Diego, CA: Plural Publishing.

tionships have three classifications similar to Angle. They are Class I, Class II (retrognathic), and Class III (prognathic) (Figure 1–9). It is possible for an open bite to be present with skeletal conditions (Zajac & Vallino, 2017).

Patients with repaired CLP are likely to develop Class III malocclusions and crossbite. A crossbite means that the upper anterior and posterior teeth are closer to the tongue than the lower teeth (Figure 1–10). If the maxillary arch is collapsed, then a posterior crossbite may develop. Anterior and posterior crossbites may affect articulation of the sounds /s/ and /z/. As discussed later, palatal production of tongue-tip alveolar stops has been associated with reduced maxillary arch width due to posterior crossbite in patients with CLP.

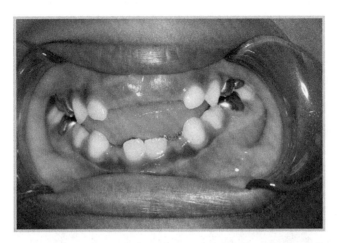

Figure 1–8. Open bite malocclusion. Note that the tongue protrudes through the space between the upper and lower teeth. *Source:* Reprinted with permission from Napoli, J. A., and Vallino, L. D. (2017). Maxillary advancement. In D. J. Zajac and L. D. Vallino (Eds.), *Evaluation and management of cleft lip and palate.* San Diego, CA: Plural Publishing.

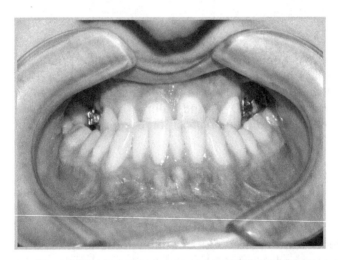

Figure 1–9. Example of skeletal Class III malocclusion typical of a patient with cleft lip and palate. *Source:* Courtesy of Joseph A. Napoli, MD, DDS. Plastic, Maxillofacial, and Craniofacial Surgery, Alfred I. duPont Hospital for Children, Wilmington, DE. Reprinted with permission from Napoli, J. A., and Vallino, L. D. (2017). Maxillary advancement. In D. J. Zajac and L. D. Vallino (Eds.), *Evaluation and management of cleft lip and palate.* San Diego, CA: Plural Publishing.

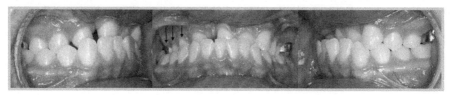

A

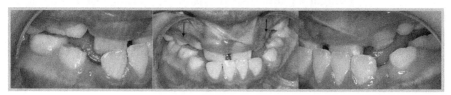

B

Figure 1–10. **A.** Class III malocclusion with anterior and unilateral posterior crossbites. Arrows indicate posterior crossbite. **B.** Class III malocclusion with anterior and bilateral posterior crossbites. Arrows indicate posterior crossbites. *Source:* Courtesy of the Department of Orthodontics, University of North Carolina at Chapel Hill. Reprinted with permission from Zajac, D. J., and Vallino, L. D. (2017). *Evaluation and management of cleft lip and palate.* San Diego, CA: Plural Publishing.

Production of the sibilant /s/ requires a precise channeling of the airstream anteriorly to produce turbulence when the air exits the constriction (Zajac & Vallino, 2017). The teeth are important in that they provide an obstacle to the airstream that creates additional turbulence and intensity (Hixon, Weismer, & Hoit, 2008). Teeth that are missing, misshaped, or rotated may result in distortion. Likewise, a forward tongue posture as a result of a Class III malocclusion may also cause distortions. When the tip of the tongue is behind the lower incisors but distal to the upper incisors, fricatives and affricates are likely to be distorted. This is called a *dental or fronted distortion.* When the tip of the tongue protrudes beyond the lower incisors, a more significant distortion called an *interdental distortion or interdental lisp* can occur (Zajac & Vallino, 2017). More often than not, these distortions are both auditory and visual. In other words, the distortion can be heard, and the way in which it is produced relative to the occlusal defect can be seen.

Patients with CLP who have posterior crossbites, lateral open bites, or missing maxillary teeth may not be able to effectively seal one or both sides of the tongue during fricative production. The escape of airflow from the side(s) of the tongue during /s/ production is called a *lateral distortion or lateral lisp.*

Obligatory oral distortions are generally not amenable to speech therapy until the occlusal defect has been corrected following orthodontic and/or surgical correction. Patients wearing various dental appliances may also demonstrate obligatory errors that occur because of the effects of the oral appliance on placement. Production errors typically resolve when the patients become accustomed to the appliance (Marino et al., 2005) or once the appliance has corrected the anatomical defect and has been removed.

Backed Alveolar Consonants

Palatalized Tongue-Tip Alveolar Stops/Fricatives. The tongue-tip alveolar stops /t, d/ are often backed to the midpalate in patients with CLP. At times, the fricatives /s, z/ are also backed. We believe that dental and structural defects such as teeth erupted in the anterior palate, oronasal fistulae, and/or narrow (collapsed) maxillary arches may cause the speaker to articulate with the tongue blade/dorsum at the hard palate to avoid the anterior defect(s). Traditionally, *palatalized stops* have been referred to as mid-dorsum palatal stops. This articulation has often been thought to be a hybrid production between alveolar and velar stops (Trost, 1981). To explain, the error is made with the tongue tip down and the blade of the tongue contacting the hard palate, a place of articulation between the alveolar and velar points of articulation. Perceptually, the palatal stop is difficult for many to perceive just by listening (Santelmann, Sussman, & Chapman, 1999). Clinically, we encourage students and SLPs to carefully observe the lingual placement, especially the middle of the tongue, to facilitate identification. The production of palatal stops results in distortion errors that obscure the perceptual boundaries between /t/ and /k/ and /d/ and /g/ (Gibbon & Crampin, 2001;

Trost, 1981). For example, the /t/ may be perceived by some listeners as either an alveolar or velar stop.

Conventionally, palatal stops have been considered compensatory to VPD (Trost, 1981). Based on clinical experience and research evidence, we believe that this error should be considered an obligatory oral distortion, especially if other tongue-tip alveolar sounds such as /l/, and even /n/, are affected. Several studies using speakers of different languages have shown that anterior structural anomalies, including reduced maxillary arch width (Eshgi et al., 2013; Okazaki et al., 1991; Zajac et al., 2012), and, perhaps, oronasal fistulae, may be the precipitating cause(s) of palatal stops in children with repaired cleft lip and palate. If so, then speech therapy to correct palatal stops may not be effective until the anterior structural anomalies are corrected, at least for the school-age patient.

Velarized Tongue-Tip Alveolar Nasals/Liquids. Similar to palatalized stops and fricatives, some speakers with CLP back the placement of the nasal /n/ and/or liquids /l, r/ to the velum. Bressmann et al. (2017) also reported that some children with repaired cleft palate back /n/ to the midpalate. Again, the reason for these backing patterns is not entirely clear but may be related to both anterior structural anomalies and/or hearing (the latter is discussed below). Obviously, additional clinical research is needed in this area.

Earlier we suggested that palatal stops be considered as obligatory oral distortions, occurring as a consequence of dental and other oral structural defects. We need to note, however, that palatal stops have also been identified in toddlers without cleft palate or palatal fistula (Chapman & Hardin, 1992). The occurrence of this error in young children suggests a developmental cause of unknown origin. It is possible that fluctuating conductive hearing loss associated with episodes of otitis media with effusion may contribute to backing errors in children without cleft palate (Shriberg et al., 2003). That is, young children who are learning an alveolar-velar place contrast that is dependent upon subtle acoustic clues may be at a disadvantage if hearing is not optimal. We need to further point out that children with repaired CLP have high rates of

otitis media with effusion. Conceivably, therefore, a combination of conductive hearing loss and oral structural anomalies
may place the child with CLP at even a greater disadvantage
relative to learning the alveolar-velar place contrast.

Other Uncommon Errors

Fricatives on Inspiration. We have seen patients who produce fricatives, especially /s/, on inspiration. Typically, these
patients have other obligatory symptoms of VPD, suggesting
that the cause may be compensatory to inadequate VP function. The child in audio sample 3.2.16 is an example of such a

case. He had repaired CLP and was receiving speech therapy.
At the time of the recording, he exhibited both obligatory
symptoms of VPD and produced /s/ on inspiration, confirmed
by acoustic analysis. Of interest, this child was recently seen
for a follow-up evaluation. At that time, while obligatory symptoms persisted, he produced /s/ normally.

Clicks. Clicks are characterized by the nonpulmonary production of stops. Typically, the tongue forms two articulatory
contacts against the palate and a sucking-type action enlarges
the enclosed space and decreases air pressure. When one of
the articulatory contacts is released, an inward rush of air produces a click sound. Some children with repaired CLP produce
clicks for alveolar and/or velar stops. In some cases, this may
be compensatory to severe VPD. It is also possible that clicks
may occur as an unintended consequence of stop production
if there are anatomical defects such as palatal fissures and/or
hyperplastic hard palate tissue.
      Audio samples 3.1.16 through 3.1.23 in the module on
Errors Within the Oral Cavity are from speakers who exhibit
various types of obligatory and backed articulation errors.

Articulation Errors Outside the Oral Cavity

Maladaptive compensatory articulation errors, sometimes
referred to as "active" errors, are those abnormal articulatory
patterns that patients learn to make as substitutions for the

targeted phoneme. In other words, the place of articulation is changed to outside the oral cavity. In contrast to the obligatory and backed articulation errors where the place of articulation is generally preserved within the oral cavity, the place of articulation for the compensatory error is shifted posteriorly outside of the oral cavity while the manner of articulation is generally preserved. The articulatory postures modify the airstream well below the velopharyngeal valve and can be an effective way to circumvent the inability to impound intraoral pressure (see Figure 1–6). Compensatory misarticulations are glottal stops, pharyngeal stops, pharyngeal fricatives, and pharyngeal affricates. The presence of these articulations, unlike most obligatory and/or backed errors, often affects intelligibility to a great extent.

Glottal Stops

Glottal stops are produced by rapid forceful adduction of the vocal folds that momentarily stops the expiratory airflow at the level of the glottis (Zajac & Vallino, 2017) (Figure 1–11). In the patient with VPD, a glottal stop may be produced in place of an

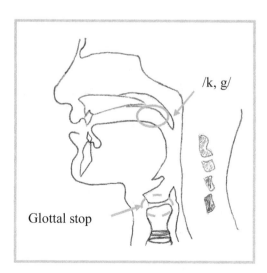

Figure 1–11. Glottal stop replacement for /k/ and /g/.

oral stop or other pressure consonant, including lingual fricatives and affricates. Glottal stops may also be coproduced with oral stops so that there is both a simultaneous oral and glottal articulation (Zajac & Vallino, 2017). The SLP must be vigilant perceptually in the case of patients articulating coproduced oral and glottal sounds. The international phonetic notation for the glottal stop is /ʔ/.

Pharyngeal Stops and Fricatives

Pharyngeal stops are produced by complete retraction of the tongue against the posterior pharyngeal wall to stop expiratory airflow (Zajac & Vallino, 2017) (Figure 1–12).

These errors are typically substituted for /k/ and /g/ (Trost, 1981). Clinically, we have also seen pharyngeal stops substituted for alveolar stops and postalveolar affricates (Audio 3.1.28 in this *Resource*). Trost (1981) also noted radiographic variability in the level of tongue retraction from relatively high to relatively low in the pharynx for pharyngeal stops. The international phonetic symbol for the pharyngeal stop is /ʔ/.

Like pharyngeal stops, pharyngeal fricatives are also produced by the root of the tongue retracting to the pos-

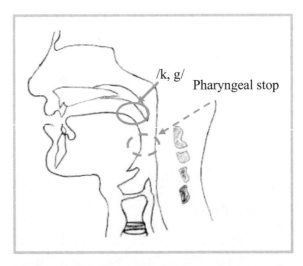

Figure 1–12. Pharyngeal stop replacement for /k/ and /g/.

terior pharyngeal wall, but unlike the pharyngeal stop, there is no complete closure but rather a narrow constriction between the tongue and posterior pharyngeal wall (Zajac & Vallino, 2017) (Figure 1–13). Pharyngeal fricatives are typically substituted for /s/. The international phonetic symbol for the voiceless pharyngeal fricative is /ħ/ and /ʕ/ for its voiced cognate.

Pharyngeal Affricates

Pharyngeal affricates are a combination of a glottal stop followed by a pharyngeal fricative (Zajac & Vallino, 2017) (Figure 1–14). These are typically substituted for oral affricates.

Compensatory errors occur in speakers with cleft palate in response to VPD. Because these errors are learned and often incorporated into the speaker's phonology, physical intervention to correct VPD (i.e., surgery, prosthetic management) will not correct compensatory errors. Rather, speech therapy will be required to correct compensatory articulation errors, the focus of which is to modify the place of articulation. Ideally, speech therapy should begin before surgery to establish correct oral placement for sounds. As Golding-Kushner (2001) points out,

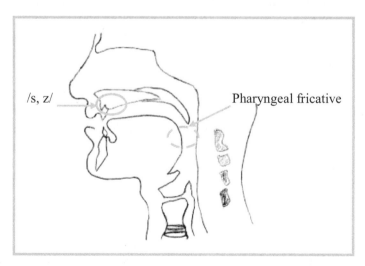

/s, z/ — Pharyngeal fricative

Figure 1–13. Pharyngeal fricative replacement for /s/ and /z/.

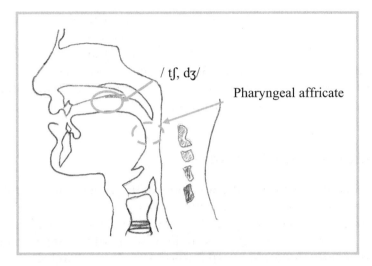

Figure 1–14. Pharyngeal affricate replacement for /tʃ, dʒ/.

these errors may not resolve spontaneously after surgery to improve velopharyngeal function. Additional therapy, therefore, will be necessary.

Audio samples 3.1.24 through 3.1.31 in the Compensatory Articulation module are from speakers who exhibit various types of these errors.

Other Unusual Articulations[1]

Some patients with cleft palate also produce unusual articulations such as nasal fricatives.

Zajac (2015) described two distinct types of nasal fricatives based on perceptual and acoustic analysis—anterior and posterior. Both kinds of nasal fricatives are produced through the nose and used to replace fricatives, affricates, and/or derived affricates (e.g., tr) (Zajac & Vallino, 2017) (see Fig-

---

[1]Although Zajac and Vallino (2017) referred to the nasal fricatives as "other maladaptive errors," until additional evidence resolves the issue, we believe that these behaviors are not "maladaptive/compensatory" in the sense described.

ure 1–6). These are learned articulations that are corrected by speech therapy.

Anterior Nasal Fricatives. Anterior nasal fricatives are produced by occluding the oral cavity and forcing all airflow through the nose. Frication noise is produced as airflow exits the anterior nasal valve, the smallest cross-sectional area of the nose. The oral occlusion can occur in the three places of nasal consonant articulation: bilabial, alveolar, and velar (Harding & Grunwell, 1998). Some children may also use a palatal place of oral stopping. The anterior nasal fricative can sound similar or even identical to audible nasal emission that is obligatory to VPD. Some patients who produce anterior nasal fricatives also exhibit nasal grimacing. In our experience, children who use anterior nasal fricatives also have VPD to some extent and exhibit other obligatory symptoms such as hypernasality and/ or audible nasal air emission during production of stops. If the anterior nasal fricative is eliminated by speech therapy, the obligatory symptoms will remain.

Posterior Nasal Fricatives. Posterior nasal fricatives are also produced with an occluded oral cavity. Although the oral occlusion can occur in the same places as for the anterior nasal fricative, most children tend to use either palatal or velar occlusion. Unlike the anterior nasal fricative, however, the velopharyngeal port is almost totally closed, which results in turbulent airflow and frication noise. Zajac (2015) has shown that velar flutter is often a component of the posterior nasal fricative, similar to obligatory nasal turbulence that might occur on stops. Because of this, the posterior nasal fricative can sound similar or even identical to obligatory nasal turbulence. Posterior nasal fricatives are often referred to as *phoneme-specific nasal emission* in children with or without cleft palate (Peterson-Falzone, 1975; Peterson-Falzone & Graham, 1990). The posterior nasal fricative (or phoneme-specific nasal emission) is a learned articulation error that is amenable to direct speech therapy. In contrast to the anterior nasal fricative, elimination of the posterior nasal fricative is usually all that is required as there are no other obligatory symptoms associated with VPD.

Because nasal fricatives can sound similar to obligatory nasal air emission and/or nasal turbulence, differential diagnosis is important. The SLP should occlude the nostrils of the child while /s/ is prolonged. If the child has actively stopped oral airflow as part of a nasal fricative, then nasal airflow and frication will abruptly stop, confirming the presence of a nasal fricative (Zajac & Vallino, 2017). Zajac (2015) also used oral-nasal audio recordings to identify the oral stopping component

of nasal fricatives (Refer to Audio examples 3.1.37 and 3.1.38).

Finally, we need to note that nasal fricatives, either anterior or posterior, are traditionally considered compensatory to VPD. The physiologic characteristics of these articulations, however, do not fit the conventional definition of compensatory in that the productions do not occur below the VP valve. More important, it must be emphasized that nasal fricatives, especially posterior, occur in children without cleft palate or other known structural anomalies. In addition, there is some research evidence to show that even among children with cleft palate, most of those who use nasal fricatives, especially posterior, do not have gross VPD (Zajac & Vallino, 2017). Because of this, we believe that nasal fricatives should be considered learned speech sound errors of unknown etiology (Zajac, 2015). Zajac, however, hypothesized that a combination of obligatory nasal air emission and/or turbulence during the emergence of stop consonants and fluctuating, conductive hearing loss may lead to the development of nasal fricatives during early speech learning. Both conditions are likely to occur in children with repaired cleft palate and may occur in children without cleft palate. Children without cleft palate who have large and/or irregular adenoids may experience transient audible nasal air emission during production of stop consonants due to incomplete VP closure (see Zajac & Vallino, 2017, Figure 8–6, p. 211). These children are also likely to experience early episodes of otitis media with effusion.

Audio samples 3.1.32 through 3.1.38 in the Other Unusual Articulations module are from speakers who exhibit various types of these errors.

Table 1–3 summarizes the articulation errors and distortions commonly encountered by speakers with repaired cleft lip and palate and VPD.

Table 1–3. Summary of Some Common Articulation Errors and Distortions Associated With Cleft Lip and Palate and Velopharyngeal Dysfunction (VPD)

Error/ Distortion	Articulatory Characteristics	Cause	Phonemes Affected
Dental sibilants	Tongue tip contacts maxillary incisors	Class III dental malocclusion	Sibilants
Interdental sibilants	Tongue tip protrudes beyond maxillary incisors	Class III dental malocclusion, anterior open bite	Sibilants
Lateral sibilants	Lack of lateral tongue contact to maxillary teeth	Posterior crossbite, lateral open bite	Sibilants
Palatalized tongue-tip alveolar stops/ fricatives (referred by some clinicians as mid-dorsum palatal stops)[a]	Middle of tongue contacts hard palate	Erupted teeth in the anterior palate, oronasal fistula, and/ or narrow (collapsed) maxillary arches[b]	Tongue-tip alveolar stops, also alveolar fricatives
Glottal stop	Quick and forceful adduction of vocal folds	Compensatory for VPD	Stops and affricates, also fricatives
Pharyngeal stop	Tongue base contacts posterior pharyngeal wall	Compensatory for VPD	Velar stops, also alveolar stops
Pharyngeal fricative	Tongue base approximates pharyngeal wall	Compensatory for VPD	Alveolar fricatives
Anterior nasal fricative	Oral stop with airflow directed through open velopharyngeal (VP) port	A learned speech sound error that may be secondary to conductive hearing loss[b]	Any fricative or affricate

continues

Table 1–3. *continued*

Error/ Distortion	Articulatory Characteristics	Cause	Phonemes Affected
Posterior nasal fricative (referred to by some clinicians as phoneme specific nasal emission)	Oral stop with airflow directed through a partially closed VP port; often with tissue flutter	A learned speech sound error that may be secondary to conductive hearing loss[b]	Any fricative or affricate

[a]Traditionally palatalized stops have been referred to as mid-dorsum palatal stops.

[b]Traditionally considered to be compensatory to VPD.

Source: Adapted from Zajac, D. J., and Vallino, L. D. (2017). *Evaluation and management of cleft lip and palate: A developmental perspective.* San Diego, CA: Plural Publishing.

■ Phonatory Disorders

The literature suggests that there is a relatively high prevalence of voice disorders in patients with cleft palate (Cavalli, 2011; D'Antonio, Muntz, Providence, & Marsh, 1988). It has been hypothesized that patients with cleft palate tend to "overdrive" their phonatory mechanism or may develop laryngeal hyperfunction to compensate for the VPD. Some individuals with cleft palate present with phonatory disorders that manifest in voice quality problems such as breathiness and hoarseness. These problems are often the result of vocal nodules (McWilliams, Bluestone, & Musgrave, 1969). The use of glottal stops has also been implicated in contributing to the development of vocal nodules in this population.

Reduced loudness is another feature of phonation that may be perceived in individuals with VPD. It is sometimes referred to as "soft voice syndrome" (McWilliams, 1982; Peterson-Falzone et al., 2010). It may occur either volitionally in an attempt to reduce perceptual symptoms of VPD or it may occur due to acoustic damping of sound in the nasal cavity. If volitional in nature, it may potentially mask hypernasal resonance. Asking a person to increase his or her loudness may unmask hypernasal speech (McWilliams, 1982) or a degree of hypernasal speech more severe than originally perceived.

Audio samples 3.1.39 through 3.1.42 in the Phonatory Disorders module are from speakers who exhibit various types of voice disorders.

Hearing

The most common cause of hearing loss in patients with cleft palate is otitis media with effusion (OME), a buildup of fluid behind the eardrum most often caused by eustachian tube dysfunction. This fluid is typically not infected, does not cause discomfort, and is fluctuating in nature. When OME is present, it causes a mild to moderate conductive hearing loss, but when resolved, hearing is restored. The most common treatment of OME is myringotomy and insertion of ventilation or pressure equalization (PE) tubes.

However mild or transient, a conductive hearing loss can have an adverse effect on articulation development and progress in speech therapy. For example, Shriberg and colleagues (2003) have reported that speech-delayed patients with positive histories of OME were more likely than speech-delayed patients with negative histories of OME to exhibit backing of obstruent consonants. As indicated in the previous sections, we believe that conductive hearing loss may be a contributing factor in the development of some traditionally defined compensatory misarticulations such as posterior nasal fricatives and, perhaps, even palatal stops. Consequently, patients with cleft palate require vigilant audiology and medical services. When managing a child or young adult with cleft palate, it is incumbent upon the SLP to obtain the results from the most recent hearing test. If hearing has not been evaluated within the past 6 months, a referral for an audiologic evaluation should be made.

Language

A number of studies have shown that preschool and school-aged patients with cleft palate are delayed in the acquisition and development of language (Peterson-Falzone et al., 2010).

They show poorer performance on measures of receptive and expressive vocabulary (Eshghi, Dorry, et al., 2017), structural complexity (Eshghi, Baylis, et al., 2017), and length of utterance. Research has also shown that patients with cleft palate may also have pragmatic deficits. For example, patients with cleft palate tend to be more passive in their conversational style when compared to patients without cleft palate. In 2011, Chapman reported that children with cleft palate did poorer on measures of early reading skills when compared with noncleft peers. Finally, SLPs also need to be cognizant of those individuals with cleft lip only. A study by Vallino, Zuker, and Napoli (2008) found that approximately 18% of the 90 patients with cleft lip with or without an alveolar cleft studied had language delays.

■ Coexisting Communication Problems

Not all speech problem errors in a patient with a cleft are due to a physiological or structural problem of the velopharyngeal valving mechanism and/or anterior maxillary arch. The SLP needs to be aware of possible coexistence of other speech, phonological, and language disorders that might otherwise be ignored by the presence of a cleft-related speech disorder that may be perceived as more salient (St. Louis, Ruscello, & Lass, 1991). For example, VPD may be implicated in a patient with or without a palatal cleft whose speech is limited and consists of vowels and nasal consonants. This problem is often more representative of a global problem of speech and language, and it is unlikely that a cleft palate, submucous cleft palate, or VPD would account solely for this problem (D'Antonio & Scherer, 2008). Another example is a 4-year-old with CLP, intermittent mild hypernasality, mild conductive hearing loss, and a severe phonological disorder compromising speech intelligibility. In this case, the appropriate management at this time would be enrollment in speech therapy for the remediation of the phonological disorder. As speech improves, the SLP will be in better position to evaluate velopharyngeal function. One last example is that of a young toddler with CLP who substitutes

nasal consonants for oral consonants as a phonological process (e.g., "noor" for "door"). This is not to be confused with
nasalizing /b/ or /d/ as a consequence of VPD as discussed in
a previous section. Based on their study of 34 toddlers (ages 6
to 39 months) both with and without cleft palate, Hardin-Jones
and Chapman (2015) reported that the production of nasal
substitutions appeared to be phonological in nature for some,
used as part of their phonetic inventory, and not necessar-
ily evidence of VPD. Specifically, Hardin-Jones and Chapman
reported that the use of nasal substitutions resolved in 62% of
the children with cleft palate that they studied by 39 months
of age without surgical intervention. They suggested that the
child presenting with nasal substitutions might benefit from
speech therapy to expand the consonant inventory and routine
monitoring before a definitive diagnosis of VPD is made. To be
sure, we have seen some toddlers with repaired CLP who use
nasal substitutions pervasively as part of a severe phonological
disorder. One child, for example, produced "nello" for "yellow." We did not consider this a compensatory pattern due to
VPD because: (a) the intended target was not a high-pressure
consonant, and (b) the child was able to produce adequate
oral pressure consonants such as /p/ in other phonetic contexts. After receiving speech therapy, this patient no longer
produced nasal substitutions, and VP function was objectively
found to be adequate.

These examples demonstrate the complexity of speech
disorders that some speakers with a CLP may exhibit. Understanding that such an overlap can exist and the importance
of making these differential diagnoses has significant implications for treatment.

■ Summary

Individuals with cleft palate can present with resonance, nasal
air emission, articulation, and/or voice disorders. Resonance
can be hypernasal caused by VPD or large oronasal fistula. On
the other hand, if the nasal airway is obstructed, the person
may also be hyponasal. Articulation errors are common. Some

errors are obligatory, meaning that they unavoidably occur as a direct consequence of VPD (e.g., nasalized plosives) and structural conditions such as maxillary arch/dental anomalies (e.g., dentalized sibilants). Other errors are compensatory or active in that they are articulatory patterns that patients learn to make to circumvent the velopharyngeal valve (e.g., glottal stops). Still others produce other types of unusual articulations (e.g., posterior nasal fricatives) that do not easily fall into these categories. Based on current research evidence, we have suggested a reclassification of some articulation errors traditionally considered as compensatory. Finally, other coexisting communication problems unrelated to the cleft condition may also be present. Best practice is centered on the SLP's thorough understanding of these problems and causative factors.

Speech Assessment

Introduction

The decisive test of a person with a communication disorder(s) is the perceptual impact of the problem. What is the impression that other speakers form when engaging in verbal communication? What is the speaker's impression of his or her own speech? This is particularly important for speakers with cleft palate, since they may present with problems that affect different speech production subsystems. Consequently, the ear is an important clinical tool for the SLP, but the SLP must develop a perceptual frame of reference for the different speech disorders, which may present in a speaker with cleft palate. That is, one must listen and be able to identify the feature(s) of the communication disorder in an accurate and reliable manner. This information, coupled with acoustic and physiological assessments, constitutes the basis for formulating appropriate diagnostic and treatment plans.

Patients with cleft palate and others with velopharyngeal dysfunction (VPD) of different etiologies often present with problems of resonance, nasal air emission, articulation, and phonation (Peterson-Falzone, Hardin-Jones, & Karnell, 2010; Zajac & Vallino, 2017). The assessment of these patients can be very challenging, but with some background information and supplementary materials, practitioners can reliably assess and treat patients with cleft palate–related communication disorders.

■ Issues With Service Provision

Prior to discussing assessment and treatment topics (see Chapter 4), it is necessary to consider some issues that deal with the delivery of services. It is to be noted that there are a small number of SLPs who specialize in the provision of services to these patients, and these providers are generally employed in craniofacial treatment centers. But most practitioners in outside settings see such patients on an infrequent basis. Their exposure to patients with cleft lip and palate (CLP) will be limited, because patients with this disorder constitute a low-incidence group. Generally, the patients with CLP are being followed by a team but may require the services of an SLP as part of their overall treatment plan (Grames & Stahl, 2017; Peterson-Falzone, Harden-Jones, & Karnell, 2010). The patients may be enrolled in a Birth-to-Three program or a local school district depending on their age or possibly be home-schooled. In these possible scenarios, the SLP will be responsible for treating their communication disorders as they grow and develop; consequently, communication with the patient's team is important (Grames, 2004).

In addition to patients with overt clefts, SLPs may on occasion identify patients on their caseloads who present with resonance and/or speech-related disorders (Gorlin & Baylis, 2009) but for whom the etiology is less obvious or even more complex. For example, some patients develop hypernasality following the removal of the adenoid tissue due to a submucous cleft that may or may not have been diagnosed (Gilleard et al., 2014). They have histories of repeated upper respiratory infections and have undergone a tonsillectomy and adenoidectomy (T&A) procedure to remove the palatine tonsils and the adenoid. Until surgery, their speech was normal, but there was a change in their resonance that did not improve following a period of recovery. Their resonance quality was altered following the surgery, and the result was hypernasality (Peterson-Falzone, Harden-Jones, & Karnell, 2001). Other patients may be identified in school screenings with hypernasality that had not been identified previously. Some may have a less obvious structural defect, which is part of a specific syndrome (Shprintzen, 2000). For example, there are patients with syndromes such as 22q11.2 deletion (Golding-Kushner & Shprintzen, 2011) who present with VPD and possible cognitive, motor, and social problems. In addition, there is another small subset of individuals who may have VPD due to a neurogenic problem such as patients with dysarthria (Ruscello, 2008a) or apraxia of speech (Kummer, 2014).

Another speech pattern that an SLP may encounter for which there is often confusion and uncertainty about VP function is the nasal fricative (called phoneme-specific nasal emission by some SLPs. As discussed in Chapter 1, the patients who produce this error do so by emitting air through the nose during the production of a fricative or affricate sound or sounds during all pressure sounds. This error is often misdiagnosed as a problem of velopharyngeal dysfunction, a structural problem, when in actuality their velopharyngeal mechanism is normal. Differentiating between this unusual articulation error and an error produced as a direct consequence of VPD is critical in making decisions about treatment.

In this chapter, we will discuss perceptual assessment of resonance, articulation, and phonation with an emphasis on those speech characteristics associated with cleft (CP) palate and VPD.

■ Assessment

The practitioners' perceptual skills are very important in the identification of VPD, but assessment is a process that involves multiple measures of velopharyngeal function, which provide physiologic, perceptual, and acoustic information. Over 40 years ago, Shelton and Trier (1976) argued that the SLP must establish a pattern among measures to identify and delineate the VPD of an individual. Over the years, several measures have been developed and used successfully for assessment purposes. The establishment of a pattern among measures remains an important part of assessment for the individual with VPD. Each aid in assessment supplements the practitioner's perceptual skills and provides sufficient information to make clinical decisions (McWilliams & Philips, 1979). Please refer to Table 2–1 for a summary of measures commonly employed.

The use of different measures will vary among craniofacial centers, but there are some measures that are preferable for obtaining information due to the type of information needed (Zajac & Vallino, 2017). For example, nasoendoscopy is frequently used to visualize the movements of the velopharyngeal port. Typically, patients 4 years of age and older will generally tolerate the insertion of the scope in the nose and produce speech stimuli to allow visual observation of the function of the velopharyngeal valve. Multiview videofluoroscopy permits the practitioner to view the velopharyngeal mechanism from several perspectives during speech. Aerodynamic study is an objective measure that detects air pressure and airflow, so that the action of the velopharyngeal port can be measured physiologically during the production of both oral and nasal speech sounds. Finally, the nasometer is another instrument that is noninvasive and furnishes acoustic information by measuring the acoustic output of speech at the mouth and nose (nasalance). Different speech samples that either contain nasal consonants or are devoid of nasal consonants are used, so that a ratio between oral and nasal sound pressure level may be computed. A word of caution: The nasometer does not provide direct measures of velopharyngeal function. Its results may be used to corroborate the perception of resonance, both hypernasality and hyponasality. Other measures that are not commonly used clinical tools but furnish physiologic information are magnetic resonance imaging (MRI) and ultrasound.

Table 2–1. Summary of Measures Used to Assess Perceptual, Physiological, and Acoustic Aspects of Velopharyngeal Function for Speech

Perceptual Observations	Description
Auditory perception	SLPs use their auditory perceptual skills to identify normal and/or disordered speech and resonance. Perceptual judgments are made while using different tests of speech sound production and other techniques such as use of a mirror placed near the nares to confirm nasal emission such as an obligatory error or part of a learned speech sound disorder such as a nasal fricative, or by alternately pinching and releasing the nares during isolated vowel phonation (nasal flutter test) to identify hypernasality (resonance disorder).

Physiologic Measures	Description
Aerodynamics-pressure/flow	The measurement of air pressure and airflow in the vocal tract during the production of pressure sounds provides information on velopharyngeal closure or lack thereof.
Nasoendoscopy	The positioning of the scope via nasal insertion allows direct visualization of velopharyngeal port activity during speech production.
Radiology	X-ray techniques used to visualize the velopharyngeal mechanism during speech. Techniques include lateral cephalometric films and multiview videofluoroscopy.
Magnetic resonance imaging (MRI)	This instrumentation utilizes electromagnetic energy to visualize internal soft tissue of the body such as the velopharyngeal port.
Ultrasound	A visualization procedure that uses ultrasonic sound waves to record movement of different anatomic structures.

Acoustics	Description
Acoustic measures	Instrumentation is used to measure the acoustic parameters of speech. Frequency, intensity, and duration are acoustic variables that can be quantified from a sample of speech. The most frequently used acoustic measure in cleft palate assessment is the Nasometer. Microphones are placed at the mouth and nose and a sound energy ratio between the two sources is computed.

A synthesis of the information collected from the perceptual assessment and supplemental instrumental measures plays a key role in the management of the individual with VPD. Best practice dictates the importance of the SLP understanding the complementary nature of these measures in diagnosing the problem and recommending appropriate treatment.

■ Perceptual Assessment

If you suspect that a patient presents with VPD, you will need to conduct an assessment that will aid in either confirming or negating your clinical hypothesis, particularly if the patient is not being followed by a cleft palate team. Most initial evaluations conducted with this population are done perceptually; however, optimal care for the individual with or suspected of having VPD requires a cooperative effort among practitioners to establish a diagnosis and make the appropriate treatment decision (Ruscello, Yanero, & Ghalichebaf, 1995).

Assessment by the SLP provides information that will help lead to a differential diagnosis, because it is based on evidence that is collected and carefully evaluated. In the ensuing discussion, an assessment protocol that will enable the collection of significant perceptual performance data will be examined. The components of the assessment protocol are listed in Table 2–2. The collection of data during the assessment and careful clinical scrutiny provides the SLP with information that is critical in establishing a correct diagnosis and developing appropriate treatment and referral, when necessary.

Case History

The first area of data collection is the complaint, and this may be a function of the family or initiated by the SLP. In simple terms, describe what has prompted the testing. Case history information forms a base for understanding the patient as she or he develops within the environment. Often, a patient

Table 2–2. The Components of the Assessment Protocol

I. Case history information	A. Complaint B. History of communication problem(s) C. Surgical history D. Academic achievement
II. Collection of a speech sample to establish the patient's speech sound inventory	A. Test of speech sound production B. Sample of connected speech

III. Analysis of the speech sample	A. Traditional analysis—substitution, omission, distortion
	B. Feature analysis—voice, place, manner
	C. Categorization of errors
	  1. Developmental errors
	  2. Obligatory errors
	  3. Compensatory errors (glottal stops, pharyngeal fricatives, pharyngeal affricates)
	  4. Other unusual errors (nasal fricatives or phoneme-specific nasal emission)

IV. Identify coexisting speech disorders	A. Resonance B. Phonation C. Fluency
V. Examine suprasegmental speech features	A. Pitch contours B. Word stress C. Rate of speech and phrasing
VI. Determine speech understandability, acceptability, and stimulability	A. Understandability B. Acceptability C. Stimulability
VII. Examine speech and hearing mechanism variables	A. Oral mechanism examination B. Speech motor control C. Hearing acuity
VIII. Cognitive-linguistic measures	A. Intellectual skills B. Language skills

will exhibit certain characteristics or problems that aid in establishing a diagnosis (Peterson-Falzone et al., 2010). For instance, there may be a report that other members of the patient's extended family were born with a cleft palate, or the patient has a syndrome or other birth defect that has a known impact on cognitive, motor, linguistic and social development. Generally, the information is obtained from the parents or another caregiver in person through a live interview, via the phone, or a written interview that is sent to the informants and then returned. The case history should also examine the following areas: history of the problem and related variables, surgical history, growth and development, communication characteristics of the patient, and school performance. Please refer to Appendix 2–A for a listing of diagnostic questions germane to these categories.

Speech Sample

A sufficient speech sample needs to be collected, so that the SLP can determine if there is a speech sound production problem, examine the extent of the problem, and assess other speech production variables and systems such as resonance, nasal emission, and phonation. We recommend that a standard test of speech sound production be used along with a sample of conversation. SLP-devised word lists can also be used and need to be comprehensive, so that a sufficient sample of speech sound production is obtained. For example, the Goldman-Fristoe Test of Articulation (3rd ed.) (Goldman & Fristoe, 2015), Arizona Articulation Proficiency Scale (3rd ed.) (Fudala & Reynolds, 2000), and Templin-Darley Tests of Articulation (Templin & Darley, 1969) are tests that SLPs commonly use to assess a patient's sound system (Skahan, Watson, & Lof, 2007). It is to be noted that the Templin-Darley Tests of Articulation consist of subtests that include the Iowa Pressure Articulation Test. This particular subtest is geared to the assessment of pressure sounds (stops, fricatives, and affricates), which is a class of sounds that individuals with VPD experience problems producing. If a practitioner is interested in developing her or his own assessment materials, guidelines are available from Henningsson et al. (2008), Ruscello (2017), and Trost-

Cardamone (2013). In using any of the standardized tests listed or clinician-devised materials, the SLP should pay certain attention to the patient's production of pressure sounds.

Responses may be elicited through spontaneous response to pictures or words, direct imitation, or delayed imitation. There seems to be slight advantage to using spontaneous elicitation in order to acquire the most accurate picture of a patient's single word production skills (Bernthal & Bankson, 2004). In addition to the speech sound test, the SLP should also obtain a 3- to 5-minute sample of conversational speech. Various procedures such as storytelling, story retelling, interactive play, interaction with a caregiver, or interaction with peers may be used to elicit the sample. Please see Table 2–3 for a summary of speech sound testing, rationales for specific data collection, and additional assessment procedures.

Because resonance problems are also a concern with this population due to VPD, this aspect of speech production can be can also be examined using the speech sample with particular attention given during the production of voiced sounds, particularly vowels and vocalic consonants. Additional diagnostic measures will be discussed for assessing resonance.

Sometimes SLPs confuse hypernasality and nasal emission. Remember that hypernasality is primarily a resonance phenomenon and nasal emission is primarily an aerodynamic event, either obligatory or learned. Obligatory nasal emission is the unwanted passage of air into the nasal cavity during the production of oral pressure consonants in the presence of an inadequate VP mechanism. Learned (or active) nasal emission occurs as part of the articulation of nasal fricatives and is usually associated with an adequate VP mechanism. Nasal emission of either type can be examined by holding a mirror under the nostrils, while the patient is repeating sentences loaded with oral pressure consonants and nasal consonants (see Table 2–3).

It should be recognized that a patient whose speech and resonance are normal might present with some visible nasal escape, so that if that is the only symptom, neither surgery nor speech therapy would be indicated. During the assessment, the SLP should observe if nasal emission is consistent or inconsistent and pay particular attention to whether it is visible or audible and/or turbulent.

Table 2–3. A Summary of Speech Assessment Procedures

Parameter of Speech Assessed	Rationale for Assessment	Procedures for Obtaining Diagnostic Information
Speech sound production	To identify presence or absence of speech sound errors and the type of errors To determine consistency of errors	To test for speech sound production, use any or all of the following: • Standard speech sound test or SLP devised • Word lists, imitated words, or sentences • Conversational speech
Nasal emission	To determine appropriateness and sources of nasal emission on nonnasal consonants and nasal consonants To determine if nasal emission is inaudible or audible and/or turbulent	Hold mirror under patient's nose while he or she repeats sentences loaded with nonnasal and nasal consonants. For example: Put the baby by the buggy Kindly give Kate the cake Sissy sees the star in the sky Joe and Charlie chew food The ship goes in shallow water Mama made lemon jam If an oral nasal fistula is present and suspected as a causative factor, obturate fistula and note any change in nasal emission

Prior to assessing a patient, we strongly recommend that the SLP review the digital speech samples included in this *Resource* and listen to the specific resonance, speech, and voice disorders, which are presented and discussed.

■ Analysis of the Speech Sample

After the response data are collected, the sample must be analyzed and the errors identified by using the appropriate framework. Please see Appendix 2–B for a summary of English speech sounds and physiologic descriptions of each sound class. First the speech sound errors are classified, and then they are categorized into the appropriate category. Generally, the traditional analysis of substitution, omission, distortion, or features is used in the case of patients with oral structural deficits such as cleft palate (Peterson-Falzone et al., 2010). However, in many cases, it is useful to employ a feature analysis, and an analysis sheet that is a modification of the work of Elbert and Gierut (1986) is contained in Appendix 2–B. It is organized by the features of voice, place, and manner, and errors can be categorized as to their function in the patient's sound system. A feature analysis can be very useful to understand the error patterns of a patient. For example, the use of a glottal stop for an oral stop would be a feature error of place (feature analysis) and a compensatory error (specific category). Both types of information are important in evaluation and treatment planning. The categorization of errors as to their function in the patient's system is discussed below.

■ Categorization of Errors

Categorization of the speech errors is vital to both assessment and treatment planning and will be discussed later in this chapter. We present here a framework that can be used to classify the speech sound errors of a patient with VPD (Table 2–4; also see Chapter 1).

Because we are dealing with a structural-based disorder, the categorization of error types will differ to some extent from those used with patients who exhibit speech sound errors of unknown etiology and do not present with sensory, motor, or structural deficits (Bernthal & Bankson, 2004; Ruscello, 2008a). The error types include developmental errors, obligatory (adaptive) errors, compensatory (maladaptive) articulation errors, and other unusual articulations. Refer to Table 2–4 for a summary of the different error types.

Developmental Errors

The first category of speech sound errors is developmental errors. Developmental errors are found in the speech of many

Table 2–4. Speech Sound Error Types That May Be Present in the Speech of Children With Cleft Palate and Need to Be Identified for Treatment Purposes

Error Types	Description
1. Developmental errors	Speech sound errors present in children that are not related to structural defects. The child may acquire the sounds or require treatment, if not acquired at the expected developmental period.
2. Obligatory (adaptive) errors	Speech sound errors present related to a variation in oral structure. Obligatory errors typically cannot be modified via traditional speech treatment. Errors may resolve when oral structure is treated via surgical, orthodontic, or dental treatment. If not, speech therapy may be needed.
3. Compensatory (maladaptive) errors	Errors learned as substitutions of individual sounds or sound classes in response to velopharyngeal inadequacy. Placement is posterior (inferior) to the velopharyngeal valve. Speech treatment is employed to modify the production of these errors.
4. Other unusual articulations	These errors include the anterior and posterior nasal fricatives. Both are produced with complete blockage of oral airflow with all airflow directed nasally. These errors are amenable to speech treatment.

patients and are not related to structural defects. That is, the patient with a cleft is likely to follow the same sound developmental process and patterns as a patient without a cleft. The patient may outgrow the errors or require treatment, if not outgrown within an expected period of time. For example, the common /r/ → /w/ speech sound error may be present in the speech of a patient, and eventually the patient acquires the /r/. However, if not acquired within developmental normative expectation, the speech sound error would be targeted for treatment. The same would hold true for a patient with a cleft palate. The /r/ speech sound is classified as an oral approximate and does not require the generation of high vocal tract pressure. Consequently, the error, if present in the speech of a patient with cleft palate, would be classified as developmental, and treatment would be guided by developmental expectations.

Obligatory Errors

The second category is that of obligatory or passive speech errors. Obligatory errors differ from developmental errors in that they are related to a variation in oral structure (Moller, 1994; Peterson-Falzone, 1988). Generally, obligatory errors are identified perceptually as distortions of specific target sounds. This type of production error is not amenable to speech treatment, since there is a structural variation in oral anatomy. For example, some patients born with clefts have a midface growth deficiency, which results in the lower jaw or mandible being ahead of the upper jaw or maxilla. Obligatory oral distortions such as lingual fronting or dentalization of alveolar sounds /s, z, t, d, n, l/ would be expected, and because of the significant variation in oral structure, such errors would not be responsive to conventional speech therapy.

As noted earlier, other obligatory errors include nasal air emission; the flow of air emitted nasally during the production of pressure consonants, which may be inaudible or audible and/or turbulent in which the air is forced into a narrowed constriction or meets some type of resistance; and reduced intraoral pressure as a result of VPD or oronasal fistula (see discussion in Chapter 1 and also Zajac & Vallino, 2017). Typically, when oral structure variations causing these obligatory errors are modified via surgical, orthodontic, or dental treatment, such errors generally resolve spontaneously. That is, functional change in speech follows change in oral structure.

Compensatory Articulation Errors

The third category of speech sound errors is known as compensatory errors or active speech errors (Zajac & Vallino, 2017). Compensatory errors are sometimes difficult to identify perceptually, particularly by the SLP who sees such patients on an infrequent basis. They are a function of VPD and often used in substitution of individual sounds or sound classes. The key feature of compensatory errors is that the patient is creating a point of articulation posterior to the velopharyngeal valve, which is not operating correctly. Compensatory errors include glottal stops, pharyngeal stops and fricatives, and pharyngeal affricatives.

Other Unusual Articulations

It is pertinent in this discussion to address separately other unusual articulation errors, most notably anterior and posterior nasal fricatives (see Chapter 1). The posterior nasal fricative (PNF) is the hallmark *phoneme-specific nasal emission* (PSNE) (Ruscello, 2008a), a term commonly used by SLPs in several textbooks. As discussed previously, this is an error of substitution that involves the channeling of air or air and acoustic sound energy through the nose during the production of a fricative sound or sounds. The nasal fricative does not occur during the production of all pressure sounds, which indicates that the velopharyngeal mechanism is functional, but it is thought there was some phonological mislearning during the developmental process. Spectrographic studies of this sound production show that it appears to be the simultaneous production of both an oral stop and posterior nasal fricative (Symonds & Zajac, 2009; Zajac, 2015).

When the SLP occludes the patient's nostrils during the production of a fricative, the person producing the nasal fricative mostly produces an oral stop consonant and no frication for the sibilant or affricate phoneme, whereas the patient with VPD who exhibits audible nasal emission on fricatives will, when the nostrils are occluded, produce frication on these phonemes because articulatory placement for these phonemes has been established. The posterior nasal fricative is amenable to speech treatment; there is no structural problem with the velopharyngeal mechanism.

Note that the accompanying speech samples provide excellent examples and explanation of obligatory, compensatory, and other unusual production errors. Speech treatment may be employed to treat compensatory and other unusual articulations.

■ Coexisting Speech Disorders

It is very likely that some patients in this diagnostic group will present with coexisting speech disorders along with their speech sound disorder (Golding-Kushner, 1995, 2004). The speech sound test, conversational sample, and supplemental tests (Table 2–5) will aid in determining if coexisting resonance (hypernasality, hyponasality, or mixed), voice (pitch, loudness, and quality), and/or fluency (disorders of speech rhythm) disorders exist.

Resonance

A resonance disorder is generally a significant problem in patients presenting with VPD. When assessing resonance, the practitioner needs to perceptually identify whether the presented resonance disorder is one of hypernasality, hyponasality, mixed nasality, or cul-de-sac resonance, and this can be a challenge. Judgments about resonance can be problematic, because resonance ratings do not lend themselves to scaling procedures that are currently used (Whitehill & Chau, 2004). In addition, phonetic contexts, adjacent vowels, and many other factors can influence judgments of resonance. A simple rating system modified from the work of Henningsson et al. (2008) is presented in Appendix 2–C. Prior to using the rating scale, SLPs are strongly urged to review the digital sound files that accompany this publication.

Table 2–5. Screening Measures for Resonance and Phonation

Parameters of Speech Screened	Rationale for Screening	Screening Protocol
Resonance	To determine the presence of a resonance disorder	Listen and rate resonance using rating scales in Appendix 2–C
	To identify type of resonance disorder (hypernasal, hyponasal, mixed)	Listen for hypernasality, hyponasality, or mixed resonance using: • Conversational speech
	To determine the degree of severity of the resonance disorder	• Counting from 1 to 10, 60 to 70, 80 to 90
	To determine consistency of resonance disorder and the phonetic contexts within which the resonance disorder is perceived	• Counting from 90 to 100 (listen for hyponasality) Use the nasal flutter test to alternately open and close the nostrils to determine if there is a difference in resonance
Phonation	To determine presence of a voice disorder (i.e., pitch, loudness, or quality)	Ask client to count from 1 to 10 Listen during conversational speech
	To identify type of voice disorder, particularly hoarseness and reduced loudness ("soft voice" syndrome) that can be associated with VPD	In the case of reduced volume, ask client to increase volume to determine change in resonance (i.e., increase in nasality of speech)

Phonation

Patients with VPD often present with a phonatory disorder (e.g., pitch, loudness, and quality) and the SLP should be vigilant to this possibility. Often times, patients with VP deficits will decrease their speaking volume, and it is relatively easy to assess. Ask the patient to increase his or her volume and document if there is a corresponding change in resonance. As previously mentioned, use the accompanying digital speech samples to become familiar with resonance and voice disorders. In some cases, the patient may engage in unhealthy vocal behaviors, which result in a voice quality problem such as hoarseness. Of importance, should a phonatory disorder be identified, a referral to an otolaryngologist should be undertaken. Please see Appendix 2–C.

Fluency

Although the expected prevalence rate of dysfluency is low among individuals with clefts and VPD (Dalston, Martinkosky, & Hinton, 1987), during the assessment, the SLP should identify its presence and describe the pattern of dysfluency and rate severity, if present.

■ Speech Understandability, Acceptability, and Stimulability

The speech sound test and conversational sample will also serve as a base to make judgments of understandability and acceptability (Henningsson et al., 2008). Understandability is somewhat analogous to intelligibility, but measurement of intelligibility for cleft palate speech has proven to be difficult when using traditional rating scales (Kent, Miolo, & Bloedel, 1994; Whitehill, 2002). The rating scale in Appendix 2–D will assist the SLP in formulating an overall impression of the patient's ability to be understood by a listener. Note that perceived understandability from the perspective of the caregiver is also obtained in the case history (see Appendix 2–A). The construct of acceptability is also an overall judgment that is related to the perceptual dimension of speech adequacy (Whitehill, 2002). A patient's speech may be understandable for a listener but may be identified to some degree as not being acceptable. In summary, these are judgments that the SLP makes and constitute an overall impression of the patient's speech production. What is the overall impression of the patient's ability to be understood by others, and what is the patient's perceived overall level of acceptability or adequacy? Please refer to Appendix 2–D for rating scales that may be used.

Finally, stimulability for speech sound errors is also a component of the assessment (Golding-Kushner & Shprintzen, 2011). Speech sounds in error are selected and presented to the patient. The patient is asked to *watch the SLP and imitate a model produced by the SLP.* Depending on the patient and circumstances, she or he may be asked to produce the speech sound errors at the isolation, syllable, and/or word levels, whatever is appropriate. If the patient can imitate the models successfully, we say that he or she is stimulable, and the prognosis for future phonetic treatment is positive. Conversely, the SLP may choose not to treat the speech sound error, because the patient may develop the correct production without intervention (Ruscello, 2008a). If the child is not stimulable, it indicates that the phonetic requisites for the sound will probably need to be taught. Generally, the sound will initially be taught at the isolated sound level using some form of sound awareness or direct phonetic instruction (Ruscello, 2017). Keep in mind that our stimulability testing is not only designed to examine oral placement, but we are also interested in the impact of stimulability on oral pressure generation and resonance. That is, is there also a change in VPD when a patient is stimulable for error productions? This would be a very positive finding for a patient who presents with VPD in terms of intervention.

■ Suprasegmental Features

Again, using the data collected (speech sound test and conversational sample), the SLP will want to assess the pitch contours, word stress, rate of speech, and phrasing of the patient. Suprasegmental variation refers to prosody, which is the flow of speech, and speakers superimpose those features on speech segments. Speakers vary pitch, loudness, and time (pause, lengthening) to give speech its rhythm or melody. Prosodic differences such as slow speaking rate, equal and excess stress, silent pauses at the beginning of words or between syllables, limited variation in fundamental frequency (F_o), reduced loudness, and problems signaling lexical (word stress) and emphatic stress (e.g., stressing a word or phrase in an utterance to signal some type of meaning) should be noted. In the case of patients with limited production capabilities, it is difficult to assess prosodic variables such as word stress, intonation contours, and inflection. Kent (1988) recommends that the patient be asked to hum or engage in reiterate speech. For example, the patient could be asked to hum a certain stress pattern of a presented utterance such as Happy Birthday or use a reiterate speech syllable such as /ma/ or /ba/ in reproducing an utterance. Kent's example of "Twinkle, twinkle, little star" would be reproduced as BAba BAba BAba BA.

■ Speech and Hearing Mechanism Variables

It is important that the SLP conduct an inspection of the speech mechanism to observe both structure and function of the oral articulators (Ruscello, 2008a). The SLP must remember that a true objective assessment of VP closure cannot be achieved through oral inspection, but important information can be obtained. Table 2–6 lists the articulators and structure/function relationships that can be observed during an assessment.

It should also be noted that many SLPs do not have extensive experience in examining the oral structures to determine if there is some negative influence on speech sound production. If there appears to be orofacial involvement, it is important to document the specific observation(s). If in doubt, the SLP should indicate the observation when making a referral for additional diagnostic observation. For example, the patient may have an oronasal fistula, which is an opening in the palate with direct communication into the nasal cavity. It may or may not have a major effect on speech production and needs to be noted as part of the oral mechanism examination.

Because of the impact of hearing on speech and language learning, it is essential to always obtain information on the ear and hearing status of patients with clefts (Zajac & Vallino,

Table 2–6. Speech Mechanism Variables That Are Examined

Oral Structure	Structure/Function	Assessment Questions
Lips	Observe position of lips at rest Observe movement of the lips	Is there symmetry of the upper lip at rest? Is there closure of the lips at rest? Is there adequate movement of the lips during the production of bilabial sounds?
Teeth	Inspect individual teeth	Are there obvious dental caries? Are there missing teeth? Are there misplaced teeth? Are there crooked teeth?
Dental occlusion	Inspect the relationship between the upper and lower dental arches	Is there a crossbite? Is there an open bite? Is there a closed bite? Is there an overbite? Is there an underbite?
Tongue	Inspect the surface of the tongue and lingual frenum Observe movement of the tongue	Does the tongue protrude at rest? Does the tongue remain at midline when protruded or does it deviate to one side? Does appearance of tongue surface appear normal? Does the lingual frenum appear to restrict tongue movement? Is there lingual fasciculation at rest? Is tongue movement during speech symmetrical? Is tongue movement adequate for production of alveolar, lingua-dentals, and velar sounds? Is tongue size appropriate for the patient's oral cavity?

Table 2–6. *continued*

Oral Structure	Structure/Function	Assessment Questions
Palatal arch	Inspect the hard palate	What is the shape of the arch form? Is there a fistula present? Is the patient wearing any type of dental or speech appliance? If so, what is the purpose and is it fixed or removable?
Velum and uvula	Inspect the velum (soft palate) and uvula	Does the velum lift symmetrically in a superior and posterior direction during vowel phonation? Is there a zona pellucida (bluish tint of the velum) when examined? Is there a "tenting" or "v" shape of the velum during phonation? Is there a fistula present? Is the uvula bifid? Is there a notch in the posterior hard palate upon palpation?
Tonsils	Inspect the palatine tonsils	Are the tonsils normal in size, enlarged, or nearly contacting each other? Do they appear to interfere with oral or nasal breathing? Does the child appear to be a mouth breather? Is the child a noisy breather?

2017). As stated earlier, patients born with cleft palate have an extremely high incidence of middle ear disease, particularly chronic otitis media that frequently results in a conductive hearing loss. Because of the often-fluctuating nature of middle ear effusion and its concomitant effect on hearing, it is very important to track hearing status, since hearing loss can be a negative variable in speech sound development. If working in the schools, the SLP can perform a hearing screening. If the patient fails the screening, he or she should be referred for otolaryngologic and diagnostic audiologic evaluations that include, but may not be limited to, tests of air and bone conduction, speech reception thresholds, speech discrimination, otoacoustic emissions testing (OAEs), and tympanometry. Based upon the test results, appropriate treatment recommendations are made.

◼ Cognitive-Linguistic Variables, Receptive Language, Expressive Language, and Academic Achievement

These data are necessary to understand the overall cognitive-linguistic functioning of the patient. The SLP may administer tests to study these areas, utilize case history information, or, in some cases, obtain information from other professionals such as the results of intellectual assessments and school achievement tests. Peterson-Falzone et al. (2010) summarized a number of research studies, and the results suggest that cognitive-linguistic impairments are prevalent in this population. As a result, the SLP needs to be keenly aware of the possibility of mild cognitive deficits, reading disabilities, learning disabilities, and school achievement problems. Communication skills exhibit significant variability among patients with clefts; however, it is clear that the population is at risk for both speech and language delays (Chapman, 2009). Data indicate that many patients show speech, lexical, and conversational delays that can persist into adolescence and possibly beyond. SLPs should be cognizant of this and closely monitor developing language skills. Early baseline assessments can provide a basis for examining language development over time and should be carried out.

■ Documenting Speech Findings

In the previous section, we described a systematic process for assessing the communication skills of patients with cleft lip and/or palate. Equally important is the method for recording the speech findings that capture the data collected during the assessment process. The recording form should provide a means by which the speech parameters are collected and synthesized in order to make an inference about velopharyngeal function. From this, reasonable recommendations can be made about the need for supplemental instrumental assessment of velar function and management. Because the information is collected and scored in a consistent manner each time, it can be used reliably to evaluate treatment outcomes and monitor progress over time.

There are several scoring systems available to the SLP assessing speech in individuals with cleft palate (e.g., Dalston, Marsh, Vig, Witzel, & Bumsted, 1988; Henningsson et al., 2008; John, Sell, Sweeney, Harding-Bell, & Williams, 2006; McWilliams et al., 1981; Sell, Harding, & Grunwell, 1994, 1999), and although not one is perfect, each provides a reasonable and systematic approach to judging speech.

A process-oriented approach to assessing the speech of patients with cleft palate enhances familiarity with the problem, provides a mechanism for consistency in reporting, reduces bias, and facilitates clinical decision making with respect to judging velopharyngeal function and making recommendations for treatment. The more systematic SLPs are in assessing and documenting speech, the more likely they will be able to draw upon their experiences to make appropriate decisions about care and optimize outcomes.

■ Summary

Many SLPs do not have extensive clinical experience with patients who were born with palatal clefts. Practitioners need to understand that these patients may present with speech disorders that include resonance, nasal emission, and phonation. They also need to understand that patients with palatal clefts may produce speech sound errors that need to be identified and categorized as to their function in the patient's speech production system. In addition, these patients are at risk for language and learning problems and frequently exhibit fluctuating hearing loss due to middle ear infections. A diagnostic protocol needs to account for these important variables and is presented for use with this population. An SLP may use the protocol to confirm the findings reported by the patient's craniofacial team or use it with a patient who has been identified at the local level. If a patient is not followed by a team, referral to a team is necessary for comprehensive diagnosis and long-term treatment (see Chapter 5).

APPENDIX 2–A

Case History Questions

■ Relevant Background and Case History Information

Purpose: To identify possible coexisting variables and case history correlates.

1. Does the child have a cleft condition?
2. If your child was born with a cleft condition, when was the surgery done?
3. Does the child have a known syndrome?
4. Is there a history of feeding problems?
5. Has the child experienced repeated episodes of middle ear fluid or infections?
6. If your child has had repeated episodes of middle ear fluid or infections, were pressure-equalization (PE) tubes inserted?
7. Does the child have a history of hearing problems?
8. Has the child had a tonsillectomy and/or adenoidectomy?
9. Is there a family history of cleft palate or known syndrome?
10. Is there anyone in the family who sounds nasal or has other speech problems?
11. Does the child appear to have problems with muscle coordination?
12. Does the child show dental/occlusal anomalies?

■ Information Relevant to Communication

Purpose: To determine if speech and resonance problems are symptomatic of velopharyngeal dysfunction (VPD).

Speech Sound Production

1. Does the speech sound age appropriate?
2. Does the child exhibit distortions on sibilants, affricates, and plosives in the presence of a dental anomaly or malocclusion?
3. Are there unusual misarticulations on specific phonemes (i.e., nasal fricatives on /s/, /z/) but not on any others?
4. Can you hear air passing through the nose during speech (nasal emission)?
5. Is there weak or reduced oral pressure on accurately produced pressure consonants?
6. Are there compensatory errors such as glottal stops or pharyngeal fricatives?
7. Is the child wrinkling his or her forehead or nose when talking?
8. Does the child exhibit any oral-motor control difficulties?
9. Is the child stimulable for improved speech sound production?

Resonance and Phonation

1. Does the child sound different than his or her peers?
2. Does the child sound nasal?
3. Does the child sound like he or she has a cold (hyponasal)?
4. Does the child sound hoarse?

■ Speech Understandability

Purpose: To determine if the child is understood by others.

1. Is the child generally understood by those who talk with him or her?
2. Is the child sometimes understood by those who talk with him or her?
3. Is the child occasionally understood by those who talk with him or her?

4. Is the child never understood by those who talk with him or her?
5. Is the child aware of any speech problems?
6. Is the child frustrated if he or she is not understood?

■ School Performance

Purpose: To determine if learning problems exist.

1. What is the current grade level of the child?
2. Is the child experiencing any academic problems?
3. Is the child receiving any special assistance for any subjects?
4. What are the child's grades in reading, math, spelling, and writing?

APPENDIX 2–B

English Speech Sounds

Place Manner	Labial	Labio- dental	Lingua- dental	Alve- olar	Palatal	Velar	Glottal
Nasal	m			n		ŋ	
Stop	p, b			t, d		k, g	
Fricative		f, v	θ, ð	s, z	ʃ, ʒ		h
Affricate					tʃ, dʒ		
Glide	w				j		
Liquid				l	r		

Vowels	Front	Central	Back
High	i		u
	ɪ		ʊ
Mid	e	ʌ, ə	o
	ɛ	ɝ, ɚ	ɔ
Low	æ		ɑ

Lingual Movement	Low Back to Mid-High Front Position	Low Back to Mid-High Back Position	Low Mid-Back to Mid-High Front Position
Diphthongs	ɑɪ	ɑʊ	ɔɪ

Syllable Structures
1. Simple shapes V CV VC CVC
2. Complex shapes consisting of cluster combinations such as CCV VCC CCVC CVCC CCCV CCCVC

Oral Semi-Vowels /w, j, l, r/
The oral approximants are also known as oral sonorants and are voiced sounds produced with minimal constriction of the

vocal tract. They do not require a significant amount of air pressure from the lungs.

Nasal Semi-Vowels /m, n, ŋ/

The nasal approximants are also known as nasal sonorants and produced with minimal constriction of the vocal tract and do not require a significant air pressure component from the lungs. In addition, they are the only sounds in our language that require an open port to the nose. This means that the velopharyngeal valve or soft palate is open during the production of the sounds.

Fricatives /f, v, θ, ð, s, z, ʃ, ʒ, h/

The fricative sounds are known as pressure sounds because they require high pressure to be generated from the lungs. The tongue, teeth, and lips create narrow constriction points through which the air flows.

Affricates /tʃ, dʒ/

The affricates are also pressure sounds because they require substantial air pressure for production. The air is forced through narrow constrictions made by the tongue in the mouth and then slowly exploded.

Stops /p, b, t, d, k, g/

The stop sounds are pressure sounds. The air pressure that is generated in the lungs is held within the oral cavity by the tongue or lips and then exploded to release the built-up air pressure.

continues

Appendix 2–B. *continued*

Speech Sound Analysis by Voice-Place-Manner   Name: _____   Date: _____

Clinician: _____

	m	n	ŋ	p	b	t	d	k	g	θ	ð	f	v	s	z	ʃ	ʒ	h	tʃ	dʒ	l	r	w	j
Prevocalic			■														■							
Intervocalic																								
Postvocalic																							■	■
	Nasals			**Stops**						**Fricatives**									**Affri-cates**		**Liquids**		**Glides**	

List Phonetic Inventory	List Errors by Categories	List Errors by Feature
Nasals	Developmental Errors	Voice
Stops	Obligatory Error	Place
Fricatives	Compensatory Errors	Manner
Affricates	Other Unusual Errors:	
Liquids	Anterior Nasal Fricatives	
	Posterior Nasal Fricatives (sometimes referred to as phoneme-specific nasal emission [PSNE])	

APPENDIX 2–C

Resonance and Phonation Rating Scale

Resonance

Hypernasality

_____ WNL   _____ Mild   _____ Moderate   _____ Severe

Hyponasality

_____ Present   _____ Absent

Mixed Nasality

_____ Present   _____ Absent

Hypernasality: perception of unwanted nasal resonance during the production of voiced speech sounds, particularly vowels, glides, and liquids.

Hyponasality: lack of nasal resonance during the production of nasal consonants and adjacent vowels.

Mixed nasality: components of both hypernasality and hyponasality are perceived in the client's speech.

Phonation

Pitch

_____ WNL   _____ High   _____ Low

Loudness

_____ WNL   _____ Excessive   _____ Reduced

Quality

_____ WNL   _____ Hoarse   _____ Harsh   _____ Breathy

APPENDIX 2–D

Rating Speech Understandability and Acceptability

Please note that Henningsson et al. (2008) indicate for rating purposes, a conversational sample must be at least 2 minutes in length.

Speech understandability—perceptual judgment of the patient's speech in relation to the level which it is understood by others.

_____ WNL—no problem noted.

_____ Mild problem—in some instances, speech is difficult to understand.

_____ Moderate problem—speech is frequently difficult to understand.

_____ Severe problem—speech is consistently difficult to understand.

Speech acceptability—perceptual judgment of the degree that the patient's speech calls attention to itself.

_____ WNL—speech does not call attention to a listener.

_____ Mild—mild speech deviation is identified.

_____ Moderate—moderate speech deviation is noted.

_____ Severe—severe deviation is noted.

3

Auditory-Visual-Perceptual Analysis of Speech Samples

■ Introduction

The preceding chapters provided comprehensive descriptions of resonance, nasal air emission, articulation, and phonatory characteristics of speakers with cleft palate and velopharyngeal dysfunction (VPD) (Chapter 1) and a systematic approach to assessing these disorders (Chapter 2). The aim of this chapter is to enhance your knowledge and skills utilizing a case-based (experiental) approach in which real-life examples are used to understand the communication problems associated with cleft palate and other problems of resonance. By reading the components of the case history and listening to speech samples, you will engage in critical thinking, apply content knowledge, develop an ability to evaluate speech within the complexity of both the physical defects and speech context, communicate these findings, and draw conclusions leading to treatment recommendations. Case-based learning is an interesting and integrative format that lends itself to an opportunity for collaborative learning and peer interaction.

Identifying the presence of a speech disorder and rating the severity of that disorder are difficult perceptual tasks for any speech-language pathologist (SLP). This is an acute problem in cleft palate, since it is a low-incidence population. In some cases, one of the perceptual dimensions may be so salient that a listener does not identify other dimensions that are components of the overall disorder. This chapter contains both audio and video recordings of a wide variety of speech samples of speakers ranging in age from 2 to 20 years who demonstrate the diverse resonance, nasal air emission, articulation, and phonatory characteristics associated with cleft palate and other disorders of VPD in the absence of a cleft. They were chosen to capture a broad spectrum of speech problems and severity that the SLP sees on a cleft palate team and that may also be encountered by the school or other community-based SLP. As discussed above, there is significant variation in the etiology of VPD; consequently, the SLP may see patients with overt clefts and those without clefts who nonetheless manifest symptoms of VPD. That is why the SLP must be alert to the symptoms of VPD, and the primary reason for including audio and video samples from a diverse group of individuals who present with the clinical signs of VPD.

The goals of these particular clinical exercises are to promote authentic case-based learning, integrate knowledge and practice, recognize the spectrum of problems that can be exhibited by speakers with cleft palate and other problems of resonance, and develop the skills necessary to effectively communicate these problems to colleagues, caregivers, and patients, and to make appropriate recommendations for treatment. The speech samples provided in the audio and video recordings can be used for both training and practice.

We begin this chapter with a description of the methods used to collect the audio and video samples and rate them. The speech samples and case studies are divided into four sections.

Section 1 consists of a series of audios that primarily present isolated examples of the types of speech features likely to be produced by speakers with cleft palate and other disorders of VPD. This will enable you to listen to and become familiar with the diverse characteristics of these speech problems before moving on to more complex case examples that contain multiple speech features. In Section 2, we move to guided practice in which illustrative case studies and audio speech samples are presented, and we provide an analysis of speech and make recommendations for treatment. Section 3 consists of audio cases for which you will have an opportunity for independent practice and to check your listening skills against ours. Last, Section 4 includes videos of a variety of speakers that simulate a more natural clinical situation and, once again, provides an additional opportunity for independent practice.

We introduce each case presented in Sections 2 through 4 with a description of the speaker's history (i.e., medical, surgical, audiological) including the results of any instrumental and imaging assessments that were performed. This history provides important information for understanding the presenting problem, establishing a diagnosis, and facilitating treatment planning.

■ Description of Procedures for Collecting and Rating Speech Samples

Collecting Speech Samples

For each speaker, written consent to be audio and/or video recorded for use in this *Resource* was obtained from the legal caretakers (if under 18 years of age) or young adults (if over 18 years of age).

The speech samples were collected from the Center for Pediatric Auditory and Speech Sciences at Nemours/A.I. duPont Hospital for Children, Wilmington, DE; West Virginia University Cleft Palate Center; and the Craniofacial Center at the University of North Carolina–Chapel Hill. All recordings were made in sound-attenuated rooms using state-of-the-art digital recording equipment (e.g., Computerized Speech Lab, Kay Pentax, Inc.) and high-quality condenser microphones.

The Speech Protocol

The speech protocol used to obtain the speech samples is adapted from the protocol developed by McWilliams and Philips (1979). As shown in Box 3–1, the protocol consists of a series of prescribed sentences and syllables containing plosives, fricatives, affricates, and nasals. It also includes counting tasks, syllable repetition, and a brief conversational speech sample.

Every effort was made to use a standardized speech protocol for all speakers for this *Resource*. However, this was not always possible, and some variability in the sampling occurred. A number of samples were previously collected as part of a routine clinical assessment over a 10-year period (well before this project was undertaken) and did not include syllable repetition tasks or counting beyond 1 to 10. The speech protocols also varied somewhat among the centers because the recordings were often made for clinical purposes to capture specific speech features, again, prior to the writing of this *Resource*. Last, for some younger children, the speech protocol had to be modified to meet the patient's age, cooperation, and linguistic capability. Irrespective of this variability, each center consistently used at least two types of sentences: (1) those loaded primarily with oral consonants and (2) those loaded primarily with nasal consonants.

Rating the Speech Samples

It is well recognized that there are several rating systems available for assessing speech characteristics associated with cleft palate. Some are more complex than others. Regardless of complexity, common to all rating protocols is the systematic assessment of resonance, nasal air emission, articulation, and phonation. Keeping in mind that the purpose of this *Resource* was to reach those SLPs and instructors who have limited exposure to the disorder, as well as those wishing to "retune" their ears, we wanted to reduce the complexity of the assessment and use a rating system that was usable and practical. The intent here was to provide enough detail to judge different resonance, articulatory, and phonatory characteristics. We believe that this process reflects current and best practice.

Box 3–1. The Speech Protocol

Sentence Elicitation

1. *Sentences loaded primarily with nonnasal consonants:*

   Put the baby by the buggy.

   Papa plays baseball.

   Give Kate the cake.

   Sissy sees the sun in the sky. Sissy sees the sun.

   Jim and Charlie chew gum.

   The ship goes in the shallow water.

2. *Sentence loaded with nasal consonants:*

   Mama made lemon jam. (listening for hyponasality)

Counting

Listening for hypernasality, hyponasality, or mixed resonance:

   Counting from 1 to 10, 60 to 70, 80 to 90

   Counting from 90 to 100 (listening for hyponasality)

Repetition of CV Syllables

/pi/, /pa/

/si/, /sa/

/ti/, /ta/

/ki/, /ka/

/mi/, /ma/

/ni/ /na/

Conversational Speech Sample

The rating system we used throughout this *Resource*, and that which you can also use for the practice exercises presented in this chapter, is shown in Box 3–2. This form may be copied and used for rating the speech samples presented in the sections on guided and independent practice.

Box 3-2. Speech Rating Sheet

Resonance

WNL/WFL[1]

Hypernasality

___ Mild   ___ Moderate   ___ Severe

Hyponasality

___ Present   ___ Absent

Mixed hyper-hyponasality

___ Present   ___ Absent

Nasal Emission

(Note: Visible nasal emission is not perceptually audible and cannot be rated from an audio recording.)

Obligatory (passive)

Audible

___ Present   ___ Absent

Turbulent

___ Present   ___ Absent

Nasal Grimace

(Note: Nasal grimace is a visible feature that cannot be rated from an audio recording.)

___ Present   ___ Absent

Articulation

___ WNL/WFL

___ Developmental/phonological errors

Articulation errors within the oral cavity

Obligatory (adaptive) oral distortions

___ Dental/Interdental

___ Lateral

---

[1]WNL/WFL: Within normal limits/within functional limits.

___ Palatalized stops (mid-dorsum palatal stops)/Palatalized fricatives

___ Velarized alveolar nasals/liquids

Articulation errors outside the oral cavity

Compensatory (maladaptive) errors

___ None

___ Glottal stops

___ Pharyngeal fricatives

___ Pharyngeal stops

___ Pharyngeal affricates

Other unusual articulations

Nasal fricatives ("phoneme-specific nasal emission")

___ Anterior nasal fricatives_f _s _z _sh _ch _dz

___ Posterior nasal fricatives_f _s _z _sh _ch _dz

Phonation

Pitch

___ WNL   ___ High   ___ Low

Loudness

___ WNL   ___ Excessive   ___Reduced

Quality

___WNL   ___ Hoarse   ___ Harsh   ___ Breathy

Additional Comments:

Impression of Speech:

Recommendations:

The three authors (examiners) (LDV, DMR, DJZ) with extensive experience in cleft lip and palate and craniofacial disorders convened for 2 days to perceptually evaluate each of the audio- and video-recorded speech samples and discuss recommendations for treatment. Listening took place in a quiet room. To enhance listening, the examiners wore headphones.

For each sample presented, independent perceptual judgments were made about the speech features of a given speaker. Samples were replayed as often as needed to make a judgment. We then compared our ratings with one another. Instead of coming to a decision about a feature based on a majority vote, consensus decision-making was applied to come to agreement about the speech problem (Shriberg, Kwiatkowsk, & Hoffman, 1984). Consensus decision-making provided a dynamic process among all three examiners in which the perceptions, opinions, and concerns were carefully considered. In cases of disagreement, the samples were replayed (as often as necessary), after which we resumed discussions of our perceptions until an agreement was reached about the nature and severity of the speech disorder we heard in the sample. As expected, we often found that more challenging cases resulted in more involved discussions. For example, and as discussed in Chapter 1, anterior nasal fricatives (ANFs) and passive audible nasal air emission due to VPD may sound very similar. Likewise, posterior nasal fricatives and passive audible nasal turbulence (rustle) may also sound similar. In these cases, we relied on the clinical assessment of the author who collected the sample. That is, the author used live procedures such as nose occlusion (see Audio Case Studies 3.3.3 and 3.3.7 and Video Case Study 3.4.10), separate oral-nasal audio recordings during production of the target to identify oral stopping as a component of the nasal fricative, and/or spectrograms (see Audio sample 3.1.15). Obviously, the user of this *Resource* cannot apply such techniques to the audio samples and may feel that it is impossible to distinguish between some behaviors based on auditory perception only. We agree. That is why we emphasize the need for additional clinical and acoustic procedures to confirm the use of articulations such as active nasal fricatives. We also found it challenging at times to identify the exact location in the vocal tract—palatal, velar, or pharyngeal—of backed alveolar fricatives. In these cases, we often supplemented our perceptual impressions with acoustic analysis by using spectrographic analysis (TF32 software; Milenkovic, 2000) to determine the relative frequency of the frication noise and to guide us in determining the location of the articulatory constriction. For some samples, some of these spectrograms are presented.

It is worth mentioning that after the in-person meeting, we continued to listen to the audios and videos many times thereafter by means of conference calls, during which time we would again independently listen to the samples and discuss our perceptions and recommendations for treatment.

A Comment on Listening to the Speech Samples

For each speech sample, an analysis is provided of the resonance, nasal air emission, articulation, and phonation characteristics exhibited by each speaker. The examiners are experts and their analyses are very detailed, but the novice listener may "miss" certain dimensions, perhaps with the more minor ones, and we felt it was important to call attention to these features. We also fully acknowledge that you may not always agree with our judgments or certain analyses, but that is to be expected when perceptual judgments are made. Consequently, we encourage you to listen to the samples several times, so that you become familiar with the type of speech features a person with cleft palate may exhibit. We recommend using a systematic approach to develop perceptual identification skills in isolating the different parameters of resonance (nasality), speech (articulation), and phonation (vocal quality) such as the one we used in this *Resource* (see Box 3–1). You may also simply listen to the recordings without using the scoring system (though not the preferable way that we recommend). To attenuate external noise and ensure optimal delivery of the different features of the speech produced in the samples, the use of headphones is suggested.

Keep in mind that these speech samples are recorded by both male and female speakers of different age ranges and speech characteristics. These varied cases are much like those seen by the SLP on a cleft palate team. It is important to consider these differences when listening to and making judgments about resonance, articulation, and phonation.

■ Section 1. Speech Features Commonly Associated With Cleft Palate and Velopharyngeal Dysfunction

Introduction

In this section, we present samples of isolated speech features commonly associated with cleft palate and VPD. These are also the types of speech characteristics that will be heard later in the case studies. The focus here is to expose you to a distinct primary symptom so that you can fine-tune your auditory perceptual skills. Even though every attempt was made to isolate a specific feature as much as possible, we recognize that some other aspects of speech may be perceived within the sample and so, when present, are noted. In order to fully be acquainted with these features, they may need to be replayed several times. Specifically, you will hear segments illustrating problems of resonance, nasal air emission, obligatory (adaptive) oral distortions, compensatory (maladaptive) articulation errors, other unusual articulations (nasal fricatives), and phonatory disorders. To make it easier to follow, we provide for each category a table that identifies each feature illustrated in the audio sample presented.

Resonance

Audios 3.1.1 through 3.1.10 contain examples of nasal resonance starting with normal resonance, which will be followed by several examples of hypernasality across a continuum of severity from mild to severe. Examples of hyponasal speech and mixed hyper-hyponasal resonance are also presented. See Table 3–1.

> *Listen to Audios 3.1.1 through 3.1.10.*

Table 3–1. Module on Resonance

Audio #	Resonance Characteristic	Speech Sample	Other Speech Features
3.1.1	Normal nasal resonance	Counting 1 to 10. Counting 80 to 90. Put the baby by buggy.	Slight dental distortions on /s/ in "six" and "seven"
3.1.2	Slight hypernasality but within functional limits	Counting 1 to 10. Sissy sees the sky. Take teddy to town.	Mild palatalization on /t/ in "Take Teddy to town."
3.1.3	Mild hypernasality	Counting 1 to 10. Sissy sees the sun in the sky. Take teddy to town.	Interdental /s/ on all segments containing sibilants
3.1.4	Mild-moderate hypernasality	Counting 1 to 10. Take teddy to town. Sissy sees the sun in the sky.	/r/ distortion and audible nasal air emission
3.1.5	Moderate hypernasality	Counting 1 to 10. Go get the wagon for the girl. The ship goes in the shallow water.	
3.1.6	Moderate hypernasality, oral distortions	Counting 1 to 10. Counting 80 to 90. Sissy sees the sky.	Obligatory dental distortions on sibilants and affricates
3.1.7	Severe hypernasality	Counting 1 to 10. Put the baby by buggy. Sissy sees the sun in the sky.	
3.1.8	Mild hyponasality	Counting 1 to 10. Mama made lemon jam.	/r/ distortion and oral dental distortion on /dʒ/ in "jam"

Table 3–1. *continued*

Audio #	Resonance Characteristic	Speech Sample	Other Speech Features
3.1.9	Mild-moderate hyponasality	Conversational speech	
3.1.10	Hypo-hypernasality (mixed resonance)	Counting 1 to 10. Put the baby by buggy. Mama made lemon jam.	Mild passive nasal air emission and oral dental distortions on sibilants

Obligatory Nasal Air Emission

In Audios 3.1.11 through 3.1.15, you will hear examples of audible and turbulent nasal air emission (Table 3–2). Recall that inaudible nasal air emission is detected by mirror testing and cannot be perceived from an audio recording.

> ### Listen to Audios 3.1.11 through 3.1.15.

Audios 3.1.11 and 3.1.12 illustrate audible nasal emission (ANE) in "Sissy sees the sky." In these samples, the spectrograms depicting the specific features of ANE are shown in Figures 3–1 and 3–2, respectively. Note the low-frequency noise that characterizes this feature.

ANE is also present in Audios 3.1.13 and 3.1.14, but you will hear that it is less salient in 3.1.14, possibly due to the lower pitch of this male speaker, which may have a masking effect. Note that the speaker in Audio 3.1.13 has mild hypernasal speech. Audio 3.1.15 is an example of nasal turbulence characterized by a salient flutter (rustle) (see spectrogram in Figure 3–3). It should be mentioned here that some authors will refer to the features in this sample as rustle, but the quasi-periodic components of the spectrogram suggest vibration.

Table 3–2. Module on Obligatory Nasal Air Emission

Audio #	Nasal Air Emission	Speech Sample	Other Speech Features Perceived
3.1.11	Audible nasal air emission (ANE)	Sissy sees the sky. Take Teddy to town.	ANE is more intense on /s/ in "Sissy sees the sky" than it is on /t/ in "Take Teddy to town." See spectrogram in Figure 3–1.
3.1.12	ANE	Sissy sees the sky.	ANE occurs on all /s/ and /z/ segments. See spectrogram in Figure 3–2.
3.1.13	ANE	Sissy sees the sky.	Mild hypernasality
3.1.14	ANE	Sissy sees the sky.	Note that the ANE in this case is less salient than the ANE in 3.1.13, possibly due to lower pitch masking this to some extent. Lateral distortions on /s/
3.1.15	Nasal turbulence	Jim and Charlie chew gum.	Definite flutter (rustle) component on two of the affricates in "Jim and Charlie chew gum." They occur on "Jim" and "chew" but not on "Charlie." See spectrogram in Figure 3–3.

Note. The specific phonemes on which audibile nasal emission and nasal turbulence occur are italicized. Visible nasal emission is not perceptually audible. Only those audible to the listener are presented in the examples. Audible nasal emission (ANE) refers to the sound that occurs when air passes through the nose; nasal turbulence (NT) refers to the sound that occurs as a snort in the nasopharynx—there is often a flutter component that when present can predominate.

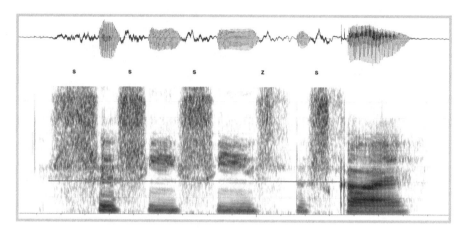

Figure 3-1. Spectrogram of "Sissy sees the sky" produced with audible nasal emission (ANE) on /s/ and /z/ segments (sample 3.1.11). Intense frication noise above the horizontal line is consistent with oral /s/ production. Less intense frication noise below the horizontal line is consistent with ANE.

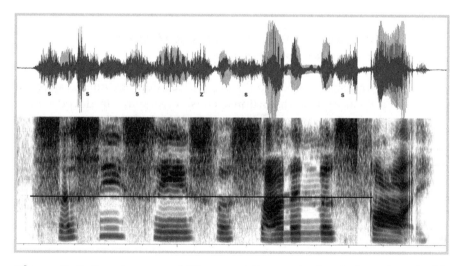

Figure 3-2. Spectrogram of "Sissy sees the sun in the sky" produced with audible nasal emission (ANE) on /s/ and /z/ segments (sample 3.1.12). Intense frication noise above the horizontal line is consistent with oral /s/ production. Less intense frication noise below the horizontal line is consistent with ANE. Note: This spectral pattern is similar to Figure 3-1.

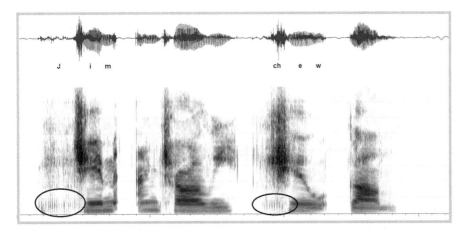

Figure 3–3. Spectrogram of "Jim and Charlie chew gum" (sample 3.1.15). The affricates in "Jim" and "chew" are produced with nasal turbulence characterized by a salient flutter (rustle) component indicated by the ovals. *Note:* Audible nasal emission as shown in Figures 3–1 and 3–2 is not characterized by a quasi-periodic component in the spectrogram.

Obligatory Oral Distortions (Errors Within the Oral Cavity)

Audio samples 3.1.16 through 3.1.23 demonstrate a variety of obligatory oral distortions. These errors are produced within the oral cavity and associated with dental/skeletal occlusal defects, maxillary retrusion, or collapse. They include interdentalizations, fronting/dentalizations, lateralizations, and palatalizations (Table 3–3).

 Listen to Audios 3.1.16 through 3.1.23.

Compensatory (Maladaptive) Articulation Errors (Articulation Errors Outside the Oral Cavity)

Compensatory articulation errors are misarticulations in which the place of articulation is shifted posteriorly, outside of the oral cavity. They are made well below the velopharyngeal valve.

Table 3–3. Module on Obligatory (Adaptive) Oral Distortions

Audio #	Obligatory Oral Distortion	Speech Sample	Other Speech Features Perceived
3.1.16	Anterior sibilant and affricate distortions	Counting 1 to 10. Sissy sees the sky. The ship goes in the shallow water.	Slight backing of /n/ on "nine"
3.1.17	Interdental /s/	Counting 1 to 10. Sissy sees the sky.	Anterior nasal fricative on /sk/ blend in "sky" θ/f substitution on "three"
3.1.18	Interdental /s/	Counting 1 to 10. Sissy sees the sky.	Mild hypernasality
3.1.19	Fronting on fricatives and affricates	Counting 1 to 10. Sissy sees the sky. The ship goes in the shallow water. Jim and Charlie chew gum.	Developmental /r/ distortion
3.1.20	Dentalized /s/	Counting 1 to 10. Sissy sees the sky.	
3.1.21	Lateral /s/ distortions	Counting 1 to 10. Papa plays baseball. Sissy sees the sky. /ta/ /ta/ /ta/ /sa/ /sa/ /sa/ /na/ /na/ /na/	Mild hypernasality ANE on /p/ segments Obligatory nasal turbulence on /t/ in "ten," /s/ in "baseball," and on all /s/ segments in "Sissy sees the sky." "ng" for /n/ in "nine" and "/na na na/"
3.1.22	Palatalized stop during the production of /t/	Take Teddy to town.	

continues

Table 3–3. *continued*

Audio #	Obligatory Oral Distortion	Speech Sample	Other Speech Features Perceived
3.1.23	Dentalized alveolar and palatal sounds	Counting 1 to 10. Counting 60 to 70. Sissy sees the sun in the sky. Jim and Charlie chew gum. The ship goes in shallow water. /si/ /sa/ /ti/ /ta/ /ki/ /ka/	Mild hypernasality Slight glottal fry

Audios 3.1.24 through 3.1.31 are examples of compensatory articulation errors, including glottal stops, pharyngeal fricatives, pharyngeal stops, and pharyngeal affricates (see Table 3–4). The spectrogram in Figure 3–4 shows the acoustic character-istics of a pharyngeal fricative. Note also the low frequency consistent with flutter or vibration.

 Listen to Audios 3.1.24 through 3.1.31.

Other Unusual Articulation Errors

Audios 3.1.32 through 3.1.38 are examples of nasal fricative errors (Table 3–5). In samples 3.1.32 and 3.1.33, you will hear examples of posterior nasal fricatives that do not have a pro-nounced flutter (rustle) quality as described in Chapter 1. The child in audio sample 3.1.34 produces anterior nasal fricatives. The child in audio sample 3.1.35 produces posterior nasal fricatives with a dominant oral stopping component and little nasal frication. Audio samples 3.1.37 and 3.1.38 are of children who also produce posterior nasal fricatives. We recorded these children using the microphone headset of the Nasometer so

Table 3–4. Module on Compensatory (Maladaptive) Articulation Errors

Audio #	Compensatory Error	Speech Sample	Other Speech Features Perceived
3.1.24	Glottal stops (in place of fricatives)	Counting 60 to 70.	Mild hypernasality
3.1.25	Glottal stops	Give **K**ate the **ca**ke.	Audible nasal emission on /v/ in "give"
3.1.26	Pharyngeal fricatives	**Si**s**s**y **s**ee**s** the **s**ky.	Mild hypernasality
3.1.27	Pharyngeal fricatives	**Si**s**s**y **s**ee**s** the sky.	Mild hypernasality. The /s/ has a pharyngeal/glottal quality (/h/-like frication). See spectrogram in Figure 3–4.
3.1.28	Pharyngeal stops	**Ta**ke **T**eddy to **t**own.	Mild hypernasality
3.1.29	Pharyngeal stops	Give **K**ate the **ca**ke.	
3.1.30	Pharyngeal affricates	**J**im and **Ch**arlie **ch**ew gum.	
3.1.31	Pharyngeal affricate / Pharyngeal affricate	"**ch**air" / "wat**ch**"	It is likely that a pharyngeal affricate is produced on /tʃ/ in the initial position in "chair." It is more definite on /tʃ/ in the final position in "watch."

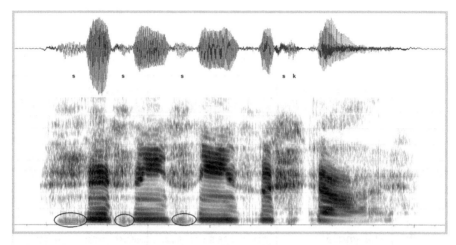

Figure 3–4. Spectrogram of "Sissy sees the sky." (sample 3.1.27). Note there is a very low frequency component in the spectrogram that is somewhat characteristic of flutter or vibration. The low frequency—almost voicing-like—is highlighted.

you can hear the separate oral followed by the nasal audio signals. While there is little flutter in the nasal signal of sample 3.1.37, flutter dominates in the nasal signal of sample 3.1.8.

 Listen to Audios 3.1.32 through 3.1.38.

Recall that the PNF is an error of substitution. It is produced when the oral cavity is occluded, the velopharyngeal port is partially constricted, and all the airflow is forced through the velopharyngeal port and through the nose during the production of fricative and affricate sounds, most notably on /s/. There is a simultaneous production of both an oral stop and posterior nasal snort (Symonds & Zajac, 2009). In particular, Audio 3.1.37 (same child in Audio 3.1.36) is used to illustrate the features of the posterior nasal fricative in "watch," "fish," and "shoe." The oral signal is first followed by the nasal signal. In the spectrogram in Figure 3–5, the oral signal shows stopping of the segments while the nasal signal shows frication of the segments.

Table 3–5. Module on Other Unusual Articulations

Audio #	Nasal Emission	Speech Sample	Other Speech Features Perceived
3.1.32	Posterior nasal fricative	Counting 1 to 10 (*six seven*). *Sissy sees* the *sky*.	
3.1.33	Posterior nasal fricative	Counting 1 to 10 (*six seven*). *Sissy sees* the *sky*.	Final /s/ of six extends into /s/ of seven
3.1.34	Anterior nasal fricative	Counting 1 to 10. *Sissy sees* the *sky*.	
3.1.35	Posterior nasal fricative	Counting 1 to 10 (*six seven*). Counting 60 to 70 (all /s/ segments).	Oral alveolar stop as component of nasal fricative is apparent.
3.1.36	Posterior nasal fricative	A "*z*ipper" A "no*s*e" A "*s*un" A "hou*s*e" A "wat*ch*"	
3.1.37	Separate oral followed by nasal audio signals of the nasal fricative produced in words by the child in 3.1.36 See spectrogram in Figure 3–5.	Oral signal: "watch," "fish," and "shoe" Nasal signal "watch," "fish," and "shoe"	
3.1.38	Separate oral followed by nasal audio signals of the posterior nasal fricative—oral stops /k/ and /d/ for /s/ Posterior nasal frication with flutter for /s/	*S*kate (3 times) *S*tore (3 times) *S*kate (3 times) *S*tore (3 times)	

Note. The specific phonemes on which the nasal fricative occur are italicized.

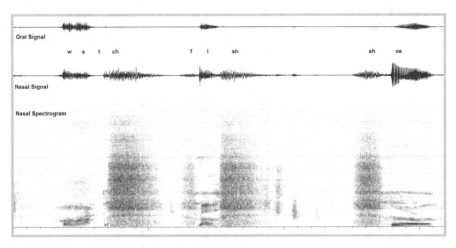

Figure 3–5. Spectrogram of a girl with submucous cleft palate and 1q duplication producing "watch," "fish," and "shoe" (sample 3.1.37). The oral signal shows stopping of the segments while the nasal signal and spectrogram shows frication of the segments.

In another example, the distinct oral-nasal features of the PNF can be heard in Audio 3.1.38. Listen to the oral stops /k/ and /d/ produced for /s/; you can hear the posterior nasal frication with flutter for /s/.

Phonatory Disorders

Audios 3.1.39 through 3.1.42 are examples of phonatory disorders across a continuum from mild to severe (Table 3–6).

 Listen to Audios 3.1.39 through 3.1.42.

Table 3–6. Module on Phonatory Disorders

Audio #	Phonatory Disorder	Speech Sample	Other Speech Features Perceived
3.1.39	Mild hoarseness	Counting 1 to 10. Put the baby by buggy. Give Kate the cake.	Anterior nasal fricative
3.1.40	Moderate hoarseness	Counting 1 to 10. /pa pa pa/ /pi pi pi/ /sa sa sa/ /si si si/	
3.1.41	Moderate hoarseness	Counting 1 to 10. Put the baby by buggy. Sissy sees the sky. Jim and Charlie chew gum.	Slight hypernasality Glottal stop on /g/ Palatalized /t/ Dentalized sibilants Dentalized affricates
3.1.42	Hoarse and strained voice quality	Counting 1 to 10. Put the baby by the buggy. Take Teddy to town. Sissy sees the sun in the sky. Give Kate the cake.	Mild hypernasality Glottal stop productions Few pharyngeal productions

■ Section 2. Audio Case Studies: Guided Practice

Introduction

In this section, we guide you through a series of audio case studies that apply and integrate the knowledge and skills essential to evaluating and treating speech disorders associated with cleft palate and other problems of resonance. For each case, you will read about the speaker's clinical history and listen to a sample of his or her speech. Afterward, we provide you with our assessment findings, impressions of speech based on our perception and key facts noted in the history (e.g., presence of malocclusion, hearing loss), and treatment recommendations. Such recommendations may include: (1) no treatment, (2) continued monitoring of speech and resonance, (3) speech therapy, (4) further assessment of velopharyngeal function, (5) surgery to improve velopharyngeal function,[2] (6) speech appliance (prosthesis), (7) otologic and audiologic follow-up. The exercises in this section are intended to prepare you for independent practice in Sections 3 and 4.

As stated in the previous section, visible nasal air emission is not perceptually audible. It will, however, be mentioned as part of the history when documented during the live clinical assessment. Only those audible to the listener will be presented in the cases presented here.

---

[2]There are several types of surgical techniques that can be performed to correct VPD. Patients in this *Resource* who required surgery underwent one of three procedures: pharyngeal flap, sphincter pharyngoplasty, or pushback revision palatoplasty with buccal flaps. The recommendation for and type of surgery selected depends on a thorough understanding of the patient, the problem, perceptual and instrumental assessment findings, and involved discussions between the SLP, surgeon, and family. The interested reader can find information about these surgical procedures in any number of textbooks and journals on cleft palate.

Audio Case Study 3.2.1

This is a 20-year-old male with repaired left unilateral cleft lip and palate. He has an anterior open-bite malocclusion that is canted up on the left side. History is positive for recurrent otitis media with effusion (OME) treated with pressure equalization (PE) tubes. He has normal hearing sensitivity in the right ear and a mild conductive hearing loss in the left ear from 250 through 2000 Hz and normal hearing at 4000 and 8000 Hz. A recent ear, nose, and throat (ENT) evaluation showed bilateral tympanic membrane perforations. He received articulation therapy in early elementary school. At the time of this visit, he expressed no concerns about his speech. He showed no visible air escape on mirror testing.

> ### *Listen to Audio 3.2.1.*

Speech Assessment:

Resonance: Within normal limits (WNL)

Nasal air emission: No audible nasal air escape.

Articulation: Very slight fronting of the palatals /ʃ/ and /tʃ/.

Phonation: WNL

Impression of Speech: Speech is suggestive of adequate velopharyngeal function. The articulation errors produced on the palatal sounds are very slight and would most likely be imperceptible to the untrained ear.

Recommendations: There are no specific recommendations for speech.

Audio Case Study 3.2.2

This is a 15-year-old male with repaired right unilateral cleft lip and palate. Mirror testing showed inconsistent visible nasal air escape.

 Listen to Audio 3.2.2.

Speech Assessment:

> Resonance: Mixed nasal resonance, mildly hypernasal (especially in nasal phonetic context), and moderately hyponasal (he had a cold and was congested on the day of testing)

> Nasal air emission: No audible nasal air escape.

> Articulation: Lateral distortions of /s/ and /z/.

> Phonation: Low pitch and mild hoarseness (possibly due to cold).

Impression of Speech: This patient has mixed hyper-hyponasality. Although the dental/occlusal status is unknown in this case, it is not uncommon for a patient with cleft lip and palate to have a malocclusion that can cause obligatory oral distortions.

Recommendations: There are no specific recommendations for speech therapy to correct the lateral distortions due to their obligatory nature and because this patient will undergo jaw surgery in the future. Continued monitoring of nasal resonance and velopharyngeal function is supported during routine cleft palate team follow-up or at the family's request.

Audio Case Study 3.2.3

This is a 9-year-old female with repaired right unilateral cleft lip and palate. She was discharged from speech therapy due to achieving articulation goals. She had no visible nasal air escape on mirror testing.

> ### *Listen to Audio 3.2.3.*

Speech Assessment:

Resonance: Within functional (acceptable) limits

Nasal air emission: No audible nasal air escape.

Articulation: Mild lateral/palatal distortions of /s/, /t/, /d/, and /n/ (palatalization was more apparent visually than during live evaluation)

Phonation: Mild vocal hoarseness

Impression of Speech: Resonance is within acceptable limits. Velopharyngeal function is judged to be adequate for speech purposes at this time.

Recommendations: No specific recommendations for speech. Monitor voice and consider endoscopic examination to rule out or confirm vocal pathology. Continue routine follow-up with the cleft palate team.

Audio Case Study 3.2.4

This is a 7-year-old male with repaired cleft palate. He has a history of having a hoarse voice and has never received speech therapy. Mirror testing showed consistent visible nasal air escape. Pressure-flow testing showed adequate but not complete velopharyngeal closure with estimated areas under 5 mm^2 and high oral air pressure during the production of /pi/.

 Listen to Audio 3.2.4.

Speech Assessment:

   Resonance: WNL

   Nasal air emission: No audible nasal air escape.

   Articulation: Slight oral distortions on sibilants

   Phonation: Hoarse/strained voice quality

Impression of Speech: Resonance is within normal limits. Speech is suggestive of adequate velopharyngeal function at this time.

Recommendations: Referral to an otolaryngologist for examination of laryngeal structure and function. Monitor velopharyngeal function and continue follow up with the cleft palate team.

Audio Case Study 3.2.5

This is an 8-year-old male with repaired bilateral cleft lip and palate and pharyngeal flap (see sidebar). He is currently enrolled in speech therapy. Mirror testing showed consistent inaudible nasal air emission.

> A pharyngeal flap is a type of surgical procedure to correct VPD.

> *Listen to Audio 3.2.5.*

Speech Assessment:

Resonance: Within functional (acceptable) limits with some mild nasality during counting and "baby"

Nasal air emission: No audible nasal air escape.

Articulation: Lateral-palatalized distortion of /s/, /z/, /ʃ/, and /tʃ/ with self-correction of /ʃ/ at times

Phonation: WNL

Impression of Speech: Based on clinical findings, velopharyngeal function is judged to be adequate for speech.

Recommendations: Given that this child shows that he can self-correct /ʃ/ at times, speech therapy may be effective in improving articulation errors. However, if dental/occlusal defects are present, there may be limits to which complete amelioration of the error is possible until the oral structural defect is corrected with orthodontics and/or orthognathic (jaw) surgery, which would be done when the child is older. Continued monitoring of nasal resonance and velopharyngeal function is supported during routine cleft palate team follow-up or at the family's request.

Audio Case Study 3.2.6

This is a 9-year-old female who underwent a tonsillectomy and adenoidectomy (T&A) procedure with reported normal speech prior to surgery. Following surgery, she became hypernasal with continued normal oral placement for her sounds. Videonasoendoscopy showed a circular closure pattern with a consistent small posterior velopharyngeal gap during speech production.

 Listen to Audio 3.2.6.

<u>Speech Assessment</u>:

Resonance: Mild hypernasality

Nasal air emission: Turbulence with definite flutter on /s/ in "seven" and illustrated in the spectrogram shown in Figure 3–6. Also perceived was mild turbulence on /k/ in "<u>K</u>ate" and "<u>cak</u>e, /ʃ/ in "ship," and inconsistent /r/ distortion.

Articulation: Articulatory placement is good; there are no perceived distortions.

Phonation: Slight hoarseness and breathiness

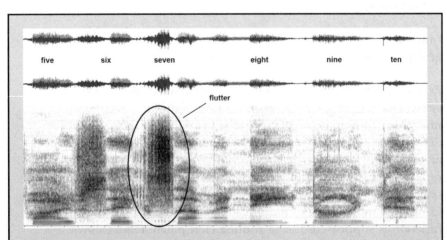

Figure 3–6. Spectrogram showing turbulence with definite flutter on /s/ in "seven." (sample 3.2.6).

<u>Impression of Speech</u>: Speech is suggestive of incomplete velopharyngeal closure, confirmed by the findings on video-nasoendoscopy.

<u>Recommendations</u>: In a case like this, we would consider the severity of the symptoms and patient/parent concerns. If there are concerns, surgery to correct velopharyngeal dysfunction may be considered. Surgical options could include palatoplasty or perhaps posterior pharyngeal wall augmentation. In some cases, a parent/patient may elect to postpone surgery and revisit this option later. Continued monitoring by the cleft palate team is supported.

Audio Case Study 3.2.7

This is a 15-year-old male with Pierre Robin sequence (see sidebar) and repaired cleft palate. He underwent early mandibular distraction for airway management. He has an anterior oronasal fistula. His dentition is marked by bilateral posterior crossbite, and he is currently wearing a palatal expander (see sidebar). Mirror testing showed consistent visible and at times mildly audible nasal air emission. Pressure-flow testing showed variable findings with inadequate velopharyngeal closure on /p/ in "hamper" but adequate closure on /pa/. He has learning challenges and pragmatic language deficits.

> Pierre Robin sequence is characterized by micrognathia (small jaw), glossoptosis (posterior displacement of the tongue), and airway obstruction. This definition has been broadened to include cleft palate but need not be present for a definitive diagnosis.

> A palatal expander is an orthodontic appliance that is used to widen the maxilla (upper jaw).

  Listen to Audio 3.2.7.

Speech Assessment:

Resonance: Hypernasality on the nasal utterances

Nasal air emission: No audible nasal air escape

Articulation: Generalized backing of alveolar sounds to the midpalate and velum (e.g., /n/) with lateral /s/ distortion

Phonation: WNL

Impression of Speech: Based on perceptual and instrumental findings, there is evidence to suggest a less than adequate velopharyngeal mechanism, but for this individual, it may be considered to be functional for speech at this time. Articulation errors are most likely attributed to his dental/occlusal defect.

Recommendations: Additional evaluation of velopharyngeal function to determine decisions about management (e.g., surgery, monitoring). The speech sound errors are obligatory oral distortions and are not amenable to speech therapy until the oral environment is improved. Speech and language therapy is recommended with a focus on pragmatic language and reducing speaking rate. Continued monitoring by the cleft palate team is supported.

Audio Case Study 3.2.8

This is a 7-year-old female with repaired left unilateral cleft lip and bifid uvula. She has never been enrolled in speech therapy. Mirror testing showed inconsistent visible nasal air escape that was mildly audible at times as posterior nasal turbulence (PNT) with flutter.

 Listen to Audio 3.2.8.

Speech Assessment:

Resonance: Within normal limits

Nasal air emission: Mildly audible at times as posterior nasal turbulence (PNT) with flutter.

- PNT with flutter on /pa/ (Figure 3–7)
- PNT with flutter on /pi/
- PNT on /ta/ and /ti/
- PNT with flutter occurs on "sees" in the first production of "Sissy sees the sky" and "jam" in "Mama made jam."

Phonation: WNL

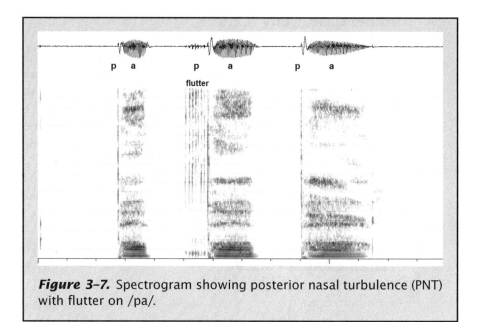

Figure 3–7. Spectrogram showing posterior nasal turbulence (PNT) with flutter on /pa/.

<u>Impression of Speech</u>: Resonance and articulation are within normal limits. Velopharyngeal function appears borderline based on the audibile PNT.

<u>Recommendations</u>: No speech recommendations as articulation was within normal limits. Velopharyngeal function should be monitored as the PNT, although inconsistent and mild, is an obligatory symptom. See, however, Zajac and Eshgih (2017) for a behavioral approach that may reduce the occurrence of PNT in some cases.

Audio Case Study 3.2.9

This is a 15-year-old female who presents with left unilateral cleft lip and palate. She was first seen by the cleft palate team at age 5, after cleft lip and palate repair. She has a history of OME with associated conductive hearing loss, treated with PE tubes. Currently, she exhibits normal hearing in the left ear and normal to mild conductive hearing loss in the right ear. She has a Class III malocclusion. Follow-up appointments were a challenge for this family. As a result, this speaker is scheduled for a revision palatoplasty and left maxillary cleft repair. This speech sample was recorded before surgery.

 Listen to Audio 3.2.9.

Speech Assessment:

Resonance: Moderate hypernasality

Nasal air emission: Audible nasal air emission on tip-alveolar stop consonants.

Articulation: Anterior nasal fricatives on sibilants, most notable during "Sissy sees the sky" and on "six" and "seven" during counting

Phonation: WNL

Impression of Speech: Speech is suggestive of velopharyngeal dysfunction.

Recommendations: Secondary surgery to improve velopharyngeal function for speech is supported. Evaluation of velopharyngeal function prior to undertaking surgery to facilitate treatment decisions is supported. Assessment to also include pressure-flow studies. Assess speech and resonance after surgery to evaluate treatment outcomes. Follow up with speech therapy to correct anterior nasal fricatives.

Audio Case Study 3.2.10

This is a 9-year-old male with right hemifacial microsomia (see sidebar). His palate deviated to the left during phonation. Mirror testing showed no nasal air emission during the production of stops such as /p/. He receives speech therapy for the correction of posterior nasal fricatives that are used to replace /s/, /z/, and /ʃ/. The nature of the posterior nasal fricatives varied with some productions having a clear flutter component while others did not.

> Hemifacial microsomia is a complex craniofacial anomaly. It is described as an asymmetrical condition affecting primarily aural, oral, and mandibular development. Features may include a cleft or noncleft VPD caused by palatal asymmetry. Hearing loss caused by ear anomalies is common on the affected side.

Listen to Audio 3.2.10.

We want you to note the following in the speech sample:

- Sissy sees the sky (Note: clear oral /d/ stops coproduced as a component of the posterior nasal fricatives)
- Words from Arizona Test of Articulation Proficiency-3 (italics/underline indicates posterior nasal fricative)

  1. tree*s*
  2. thi*s*
  3. chair
  4. green
  5. watch
  6. thumb

7. mouth
8. zipper (flutter)
9. nose (flutter)
10. sun
11. house
12. step (flutter)
13. nest
14. carrot
15. books

Speech Assessment:

Resonance: Normal resonance

Nasal air emission: No obligatory nasal air escape (only part of the posterior nasal fricatives).

Articulation: Unusual articulation characterized by posterior nasal fricatives with variable flutter during production of /s/, /z/, and /ʃ/, / tʃ/ produced normally; was stimulable for oral /s/ in isolation facilitated by prolonging release of /t/.

Phonation: WNL

Impression of Speech: The posterior nasal fricatives are learned articulatory patterns of speech. Normal resonance and adequate sound production on all other oral consonants are suggestive of adequate velopharyngeal function.

Recommendations: Continued speech therapy to eliminate posterior nasal fricatives and correct sibilant production is recommended.

Audio Case Study 3.2.11

(*Note.* This case is also presented in Video 3.4.10.)

This is an 8-year-old female referred to the cleft palate team because of concerns about nasal resonance. Oral examination revealed a submucous cleft palate on the basis of a palpable notch in the posterior hard palate, with a deep furrow in the midline with soft palate elevation. There was also a translucent zone in the midline of the soft palate. The uvula has a midline furrow, but a definitive bifid uvula could not be visualized. She has a large anterior open bite as a result of a thumbsucking habit. She has low muscle tone. Pressure-flow studies showed nasal and oral air pressures to be equal, indicative of velopharyngeal inadequacy.

> *Listen to Audio 3.2.11.*

Speech Assessment:

Resonance: Mild hypernasality

Nasal air emission: Mild audible nasal air emission

Articulation: Interdentalized sibilants and an unusual gr/w substitution in the word "wagon."

Phonation: No hoarse voice quality perceived.

Impression of Speech: Speech is suggestive of VPD on the basis of hypernasality, confirmed by the results from pressure-flow testing.

Recommendations: In this case, we would support further assessment of velopharyngeal function using imaging procedures (i.e., videonasoendoscopy and/or multiview videofluoroscopy) to facilitate treatment planning that may include surgical repair of the submucous cleft palate. Improvement for the interdentalized sibilants will not be possible until the open-bite occlusal defect is corrected. Referral for orthodontic treatment for the open bite is recommended.

Audio Case Study 3.2.12

This is an 8-year-old female who presents with a small fistula in the soft palate. She was diagnosed with a malignant oral tumor and underwent surgery, which resulted in a large lesion that included removal of portions of the soft and hard palate. She underwent a repair that resulted in complete closure with the exception of the small fistula.

 Listen to Audio 3.2.12.

Speech Assessment:

Resonance: Very mild hypernasality on "eight" but otherwise considered to be within acceptable limits

Nasal air emission: No audible nasal air escape

Articulation: Articulation is within normal limits; there are no oral placement errors.

Phonation: Mild hard glottal attack on the vowels during counting from 80 to 85 and even the first 60, although not extreme. Of note, the acoustic wave supported this perception as shown by an increased amplitude at the beginning of the vowels.

Impression of Speech: Speech is judged to be within acceptable limits. This child, after ablative surgery of the palate, is doing well.

Recommendations: Although there is no specific treatment for hypernasal resonance recommended at this time, monitoring of resonance and velopharyngeal function is supported.

Audio Case Study 3.2.13

This is an almost 13-year-old female with a profound, rising to mild mixed hearing loss in the right ear and severe, rising to mild mixed hearing loss in the left ear for which she wears bilateral hearing aids. She has a history of speech therapy. She is a singer who indicated satisfaction with her speech and that her resonance does not have an impact on her singing voice.

> ***Listen to Audio 3.2.13.***

Speech Assessment:

 Resonance: Moderate hypernasality

 Nasal air emission: No audible nasal air escape

 Articulation: WNL; there are no oral placement errors

 Phonation: WNL

Impression of Speech: The hypernasality and unusual resonance quality is attributed to this patient's severe hearing loss. It is interesting to note that her articulation appears not to be affected by the hearing impairment.

Recommendations: Given that the patient has no concerns about speech, there are no specific recommendations to treat her hypernasality. The patient is encouraged to return to the cleft palate team should she, at any time, have concerns about nasal resonance. Routine audiological evaluations and hearing aid checks are supported.

Audio Case Study 3.2.14

This is a 19-year-old female with muscular dystrophy and flaccid dysarthria. Pressure-flow test results showed evidence of velopharyngeal dysfunction.

 Listen to Audio 3.2.14.

Speech Assessment:

    Resonance: Moderate hypernasality

    Nasal air emission: No audible nasal air escape

    Articulation: Imprecise articulation on /s/, /sk/ in 60 to 70 counting and other speech sound distortions that are attributed to the flaccid dysarthria

    Phonation: WNL

Impression of Speech: The hypernasality is suggestive of VPD, further confirmed by the pressure-flow results. The resonance feature and imprecise articulation are characteristics of dysarthria. Her overall intelligibility is judged to be satisfactory.

Recommendations: Referral for the fitting of a palatal lift due to the consistent leakage of air flow during pressure-flow testing. The rationale is to improve resonance and support her respiratory control for speech due to the flaccid dysarthria.

Audio Case Study 3.2.15

This is a 12-year-old female without cleft palate. She has a history of hypernasal speech after tonsillectomy and adenoidectomy at 6 years of age. Oral examination showed limited velar movement during phonation. Pressure-flow testing showed estimated velopharyngeal areas that ranged from 17 to 97 mm^2 during various speech samples (areas under 5 mm^2 are considered adequate).

> ### *Listen to Audio 3.2.15.*

Speech Assessment:

    Resonance: Moderate-severe hypernasality

    Nasal air emission: Audible nasal air emission

    Articulation: Slight interdental lisp

    Phonation: WNL

Impression of Speech: Speech symptoms including moderate-severe hypernasality are consistent with VPD, further confirmed by pressure-flow test results.

Recommendations: Physical management, either surgery or obturator bulb appliance, to improve velopharyngeal function for speech. Postoperative speech assessment is recommended to monitor treatment outcomes.

Audio Case Study 3.2.16

This is a 6-year-old male with repaired right unilateral cleft lip and palate. Oral examination showed a Passavant's ridge. Pressure-flow testing showed inadequate velopharyngeal closure as evidenced by nasal airflow exceeding 250 mL/s during /pi/. He is enrolled in speech therapy.

 Listen to Audio 3.2.16.

Speech Assessment:

Resonance: Moderately hypernasality

Nasal air emission: Audible nasal emission

Articulation: WNL except for /s/ produced on inspiration; stimulable for oral /s/ on exhalation by occluding nose and prolonging release of /t/

Phonation: Reduced loudness

Impression of Speech: Speech is suggestive of VPD, confirmed by pressure-flow test results.

Recommendations: Consider further assessment of the velopharyngeal mechanism using imaging in order to determine a treatment plan to improve velopharyngeal function for speech. Continue speech therapy for articulation, not nasality.

Audio Case Study 3.2.17

This is a 14-year-old male with repaired bilateral cleft lip and palate. His lip was repaired at 3 months, the palate repaired at 1 year, and maxillary alveolar cleft repair at 9 years. He has a history of OME treated with PE tubes. The most recent audiogram revealed normal hearing sensitivity, bilaterally. He has a Class III malocclusion. He received speech therapy in elementary school and no longer receives this service. This teen indicated during several team visits that he is not interested in improving his speech. He did not want to pursue imaging procedures to assess velopharyngeal function and did not want surgery. His family supported his decision.

Listen to Audio 3.2.17.

Speech Assessment:

Resonance: Moderate hypernasality

Nasal air emission: Audible nasal emission most noticeable on sibilants ("sissy sees the sky"). Weak pressure consonants perceived.

Articulation: Oral distortions characterized by palatalization of sibilants and the tip-alveolar stop consonant /t/ most likely associated with dentition and occlusal status.

Phonation: WNL

Impression of Speech: Speech is suggestive of VPD.

Recommendations: Although surgery to correct VPD is recommended, the team has to acknowledge and respect the patient, and his family has the right to make the decision regarding his care. In this case, and at this time, they elected not to pursue further assessment of velopharyngeal function or surgical intervention. The team and family agreed to continue to revisit these recommendations in the future should this patient be interested in improving his speech. Continued team follow-up is supported.

Audio Case Study 3.2.18

This is a 6-year-old male with a complete cleft lip and palate. The lip was repaired at 3 months and the palate repaired at 13 months. He is currently receiving speech therapy.

 Listen to Audio 3.2.18.

Speech Assessment:

    Resonance: Moderate hypernasality

    Nasal air emission: No audible nasal air escape

    Articulation: Compensatory articulation errors characterized by glottal stops. Note that the production of oral stops and most of the glottal stop substitutions are in place of fricatives.

    Phonation: Excess vocal loudness

Impression of Speech: The errors present in this child's conversational speech compromise his intelligibility. Speech findings are suggestive of VPD.

Recommendations: Continued speech therapy for the elimination of the compensatory articulations and establishment of correct oral placement for sounds is supported. Imaging of the velopharyngeal mechanism focusing on oral consonants will be required.

Audio Case Study 3.2.19

(*Note.* This child is also shown in Video 3.4.15. He is younger in this audio example than he is in the video.)

This is a 3.5-year-old male with repaired left unilateral cleft lip and palate who presented to the cleft palate team for the first time. He was internationally adopted at age 3, after cleft lip and palate repair. He is currently receiving speech therapy.

> *Listen to Audio 3.2.19.*

Speech Assessment:

Resonance: Mild hypernasality

Nasal air emission: Audible nasal air emission on sibilants /s/ and /ʃ/

Articulation: Developmental d/dʒ and t/ʃ substitutions, and h/p.

Phonation: High pitch overall with an extreme range (Note: Acoustic measurements not shown indicate frequency of some vowels approaching 475 Hz)

Other: One instance of inhalation between "to" and "town" in "Take Teddy to town"

Impression of Speech: Based on the presence of hypernasality, VPD is suspected. The articulation errors are developmental in nature and unrelated to the cleft palate. The inspiration perceived on /t/ is unusual.

Recommendations: Further assessment of velopharyngeal function for speech using imaging procedures such as multiview videofluoroscopy and/or videonasoendoscopy and pressure-flow studies to determine a plan for treatment. Continue speech therapy for articulation.

Audio Case Study 3.2.20

This is a 4-year-old male with repaired left unilateral cleft lip and palate who presented to the cleft palate team for the first time. He was internationally adopted at age 3, after lip and palate repair. The palate was repaired at 19 months. A revision palatoplasty was recently done at which time PE tubes were inserted to treat OME.

 Listen to Audio 3.2.20.

Speech Sample (to assist in listening)

- Counting from 1 to 5
- Baby buggy
- Chewing gum
- Get wagon
- Give cake
- Lemon jam
- Shallow ship
- Sister Sue
- Take Teddy

Speech Assessment:

Resonance: Moderate hypernasality

Nasal air emission: Audible nasal air emission

Articulation: y/l substitution in "lemon" and stopping errors including: t/s in "sister," d/g in "gum."

Phonation: WNL

Impression of Speech: Speech is suggestive of VPD, for which further study is warranted. Some developmental errors coexist.

Recommendations: Further assessment of velopharyngeal function for speech using imaging procedures such as multiview videofluoroscopy and/or videonasoendoscopy and pressure-flow studies to determine a plan for treatment to improve velopharyngeal function. Continued speech therapy for the correction of articulation errors unrelated to VPD is supported.

■ Section 3. Audio Case Studies: Independent Practice

Introduction

In this section, you will have the opportunity for independent practice in listening to and analyzing a variety of communication disorders with increasing complexity associated with cleft palate and other problems of VPD. Begin by reading the information from the case history. You will see that, with few exceptions, the histories are detailed. This detail encourages a larger focus on a complex problem rather than focusing on a single solitary aspect of it (e.g., resonance), which is important in making a diagnosis and deciding on a treatment plan. After you read the history, listen to the speech sample and identify the salient features of the speaker's speech, giving consideration of causative factors leading to the speech disorder. It is helpful to think about the information presented in the case history (i.e., presence of a malocclusion, history of otitis media with effusion [OME]) that will assist in the differential diagnosis. Synthesize your findings to formulate a clinical impression and consider recommendations for management. As you read the case studies and listen to the samples, you will become increasingly engaged with the nuances of differential diagnosis.

The samples may be replayed as often as needed. Afterward, you will then have the opportunity to compare your listening skills and diagnostic and treatment expertise with ours found in Appendix A at the end of this book. Do not be discouraged to find that your analysis does not always match ours. Even SLPs with years of experience in cleft palate do not agree completely about the nature of every speech error. If you find disagreements or miss a feature, you should relisten to the sample(s) for resolution.

Reminder: When listening to these audios, remember that inaudible nasal air emission is detected by mirror testing and cannot be perceived from an audio recording. There may be instances, however, when you perceive audible or turbulent nasal air emission. Further remember that obligatory nasal air emission and nasal turbulence (rustle) may sound similar or identical to nasal fricatives. Thus, an accurate differential diagnosis may not be possible in some cases based solely on the audio samples.

Audio Case Study 3.3.1

This is a 20-year-old male with repaired bilateral cleft lip and palate.

Case History

Surgical: Tracheostomy in the newborn period for subglottic stenosis and was decannulated at 1 year of age. Lip repair at 9 months, palate repair at 19 months, and a superiorly based pharyngeal flap to correct VPD at age 5 years. He has a history of OME treated with PE tubes.

Dental: Severe skeletal Class III malocclusion with open bite. This patient is currently preparing for maxillary advancement (LeFort I osteotomy) using distraction osteogenesis (MADO) (see sidebar).

> Maxillary advancement using distraction osteogenesis (MADO) is a surgical technique involving an osteotomy of the maxilla similar to conventional maxillary advancement. Distractors are attached to the facial skeleton and gradually adjusted to advance the upper jawbone approximately 1 mm each day until the maxilla is in the desired position. Once new bone has consolidated (mineralize and harden), the distractors are removed.

Hearing: An audiological evaluation completed at the time of this assessment showed normal hearing sensitivity, bilaterally.

Speech Therapy: History of speech therapy in elementary school. During his clinical visit, this young adult expressed no concerns about his speech.

Listen to Audio 3.3.1.

Audio Case Study 3.3.2

This is a 12-year-old male with repaired left cleft lip and palate and history of left maxillary collapse. Mirror testing showed no visible nasal air emission. He has no history of speech therapy.

 Listen to Audio 3.3.2.

Audio Case Study 3.3.3

This is a 7-year-old male with repaired bilateral cleft lip and palate.

Case History

<u>Surgical</u>: Lip repair at 3 months, palate at 14 months, and a sphincter pharyngoplasty (see sidebar) at age 6 years.

> A sphincter pharyngoplasty is a type of surgical procedure to correct VPD.

<u>Dental</u>: Narrow premaxillary segment that will require correction.

> **Listen to Audio 3.3.3.** *Note.* In this audio, you will hear the SLP providing speech prompts.

Audio Case Study 3.3.4

This is a 9-year-old male with Stickler syndrome (see sidebar) and repaired cleft palate. His features include mandibular hypoplasia and myopia (near-sightedness), for which he wears glasses, and hearing loss. Throughout the years, the caretaker had considered this child's speech to be acceptable even though hypernasality had been documented during previous routine team visits. More recently, she expressed concerns about the child's nasality.

> Stickler syndrome is a genetic disorder characterized by a flattened midface, micrognathia, wide nasal bridge, cleft palate (which may or may not be present), hearing loss, eye abnormalities, and joint problems.

Case History

Surgical: Mandibular distraction osteogenesis to improve the airway at 2 months and cleft palate repair at 10 months

Dental: Class II malocclusion

Hearing: An audiological evaluation completed at the time of this assessment showed a mild to moderate sensorineural hearing loss (SNHL) in the right ear and a mild to moderate mixed hearing loss 250 to 6000 Hz sloping to profound at 8000 Hz in the left ear. The family is not interested in pursuing amplification.

Speech Therapy: Received private speech therapy as a toddler and was discharged from this service by the time he entered school.

 Listen to Audio 3.3.4.

Audio Case Study 3.3.5

This is an 11-year-old female with 22q11.2 deletion syndrome (see sidebar) who was referred to the cleft palate team due to concerns regarding hypernasality. She does not have a cleft palate.

> 22q11.2 deletion syndrome is a genetic disorder with variable expression. Clinical features include facial anomalies, palatal anomalies, cardiac anomalies, hypotonia, learning challenges, and communication impairment, including resonance, articulation, and language problems. The symptoms can vary.

Case History

<u>Surgical</u>: None to date

<u>Dental</u>: Class I molar relationship

<u>Hearing</u>: An audiological evaluation completed at the time of this assessment showed normal hearing, bilaterally.

<u>Speech Therapy</u>: She has a history of speech and language therapy, and experiences some learning challenges. Based on the Individualized Educational Program (IEP), the current focus of speech therapy is on the remediation of /k, g/ and /s/.

<u>Pressure-Flow Studies</u>: Findings were suggestive of variable velopharyngeal closure ranging from complete to incomplete closure.

Listen to Audio 3.3.5.

Audio Case Study 3.3.6

This is an 11-year-old male with a repaired left unilateral cleft lip and palate. This was his first visit with the cleft palate team.

Case History

<u>Surgical</u>: The cleft lip and palate were repaired but a left maxillary cleft remains and requires repair.

<u>Dental</u>: Mixed dentition and dental crowding. Class III relationship with anterior and bilateral posterior crossbite. The palate appears short in the anterior-posterior dimension.

<u>Hearing</u>: History of otitis media with effusion treated with PE tubes. Mild low-frequency conductive hearing loss in the left ear and normal hearing in the right ear.

<u>Speech Therapy</u>: Currently enrolled in speech therapy for correction of /s/ and /z/.

 Listen to Audio 3.3.6.

Audio Case Study 3.3.7

This 4-year-old female was referred by her otolaryngologist for an assessment of velopharyngeal function for speech.

Case History

<u>Surgical</u>: No surgical surgery

<u>Hearing</u>: An audiological evaluation completed at the time of this assessment showed normal hearing, bilaterally.

<u>Speech Therapy</u>: The child has a history of speech therapy to correct articulation errors.

Listen to Audio 3.3.7.

Audio Case Study 3.3.8

This is a 15-year-old male with popliteal pterygium syndrome (see sidebar), cleft palate, lip pits on the lower lip, and left choanal atresia with recurrent nasal congestion. There is a fistula at the junction of the hard and soft palate approximately 2 mm wide and 3 to 4 mm in length. He has a history of OME treated with PE tubes.

> Popliteal pterygium syndrome is a genetic disorder that involves clefting, lip pits, and various digital anomalies.

Case History

<u>Surgical</u>: Palate repair at 8 months. The choanal atresia was repaired, resulting in improved airflow through the nose.

<u>Dental</u>: Deep vertical overbite

<u>Hearing</u>: An audiological evaluation completed at the time of this assessment showed that hearing sensitivity is essentially within normal limits for the left ear, with a slight hearing loss noted at 250 and 6000 Hz, and a slight conductive hearing loss present from 1000 to 2000 Hz in the right ear.

<u>Videonasoendoscopic Assessment</u>: Videonasoendoscopy showed a coronal pattern of velopharyngeal movement with a large central gap. These findings were discussed with the caregiver and patient, who indicated that he is not currently interested in treatment to correct his VPD.

 Listen to Audio 3.3.8.

Audio Case Study 3.3.9

This is a 17-year-old female with repaired right unilateral cleft lip and palate. She has a history of maxillary advancement, resulting in increased nasality.

Case History

<u>Surgical</u>: Maxillary advancement to correct malocclusion, after which she reported experiencing occasional nasal reflux.

<u>Oral Examination</u>: A well-formed Passavant's ridge was observed.

<u>Pressure Flow Studies</u>: Findings showed estimated velopharyngeal areas ranging from 12 to 38 mm^2 depending upon the speech sample.

Listen to Audio 3.3.9.

Audio Case Study 3.3.10

This is a 6-year-old female with repaired bilateral cleft lip and palate. She has maxillary alveolar clefts that will be repaired. She has a history of OME and hearing loss.

Case History

Surgical: Lip repair at 4 months and palate repair at 11 months

Dental: Class III bilateral posterior crossbite

Hearing: An audiological evaluation completed at the time of this assessment showed a mild conductive hearing loss at 250 and 500 Hz rising to normal hearing from 1000 to 8000 Hz, bilaterally.

Speech Therapy: History of speech therapy beginning with Early Intervention. She continues to receive this service through the school district.

Listen to Audio 3.3.10.

Audio Case Study 3.3.11

(*Note.* This case is also presented in Video 3.4.6.)

This is an 18-year-old female with repaired left unilateral cleft lip and palate. She first presented to the cleft palate team at age 7.

Case History

(Additional information about this young adult's background is provided in the history for Video 3.4.6.)

<u>Surgical</u>: Palate repaired at 12 months

<u>Dental</u>: She is in active orthodontics and has a Class I molar relationship.

<u>Hearing</u>: She has a history of OME and hearing loss.

<u>Pressure-Flow Studies</u>: Findings showed estimated velopharyngeal orifice areas that exceeded 20 mm^2, consistent with inadequate velopharyngeal closure.

<u>Imaging Studies</u>: Multiview videofluoroscopy and videonasoendoscopy confirmed VPD.

<u>Speech Therapy</u>: No known history of speech therapy

Listen to Audio 3.3.11.

Audio Case Study 3.3.12

This is an 8-year-old female with Stickler syndrome and repaired isolated cleft palate. She reported that her classmates have a difficult time understanding her. It is worth noting that for the past several years, this child had been scheduled for instrumental assessment of velopharyngeal function, but the parents did not keep the appointments.

Case History

Surgical: Palate repaired at 11 months. PE tubes to manage OME were inserted at the time of palate repair. Tubes were replaced at age 5 years.

Dental: Mixed dentition with a left posterior crossbite and Class I occlusion

Hearing: An audiological evaluation completed at the time of this assessment showed normal hearing, bilaterally.

Pressure-Flow Studies: Findings showed estimated VP areas of 7.2 mm^2 on /p/ in "hamper" with complete overlap of oral pressure, nasal pressure, and nasal airflow during /mp/ segments. Recorded mean nasal airflow rate on /p/ in syllables was 149 mL/s. These results are consistent with marginal velar closure.

Speech Therapy: She has never been enrolled in speech therapy.

 Listen to Audio 3.3.12.

Audio Case Study 3.3.13

This is a 13-year-old male with Klippel-Feil syndrome (see sidebar) and repaired left unilateral cleft lip and palate who was first seen by the team at age 7 years. He also has microcephaly, hearing loss for which he wears hearing aids, and learning challenges. He also wears glasses. He has limited nasal air flow through both nostrils.

> Klippel-Feil syndrome is a bone disorder characterized by the fusion of two or more cervical vertebrae and short neck, and limited range of neck motion. Additional clinical features include cleft palate, hearing loss, and other skeletal and body defects.

Case History

Surgical: Lip and palate surgery was done elsewhere. The timing of surgery is unknown.

Dental: Class III molar relationship and mixed dentition. He wears a maxillary holding appliance.

Hearing: An audiological evaluation completed at the time of this assessment showed a moderately severe rising to essentially slight conductive hearing loss in the right ear and a moderate rising to essentially mild conductive hearing loss in the left ear. He wears binaural hearing aids.

Speech Therapy: He has a history of speech and language therapy, beginning with Early Intervention. He continues to receive this service at school. The mother reported that the focus of treatment is on rate reduction.

Listen to Audio 3.3.13.

Audio Case Study 3.3.14

(*Note.* This child is also shown in Video 3.4.12.)

This is an almost 8-year-old male with repaired bilateral cleft lip and palate who was internationally adopted at 15 months of age. He has a history of OME and hearing loss.

Case History

Surgical: Cleft lip was repaired in the country of birth prior to adoption. Palate repair at 17 months after he joined his family. PE tubes inserted at the time of palate repair.

Dental: Early mixed dentition. Skeletal Class III. There is an anterior crossbite and a left crossbite in the canine and first molar region.

Hearing: An audiological evaluation completed at the time of this assessment showed a mild low-frequency conductive hearing loss, bilaterally.

Speech Therapy: Started speech therapy through Early Intervention and is currently receiving treatment at school and hospital-based programs to correct articulation errors.

Pressure-Flow Studies: Findings showed estimated VP areas exceeding that of 20 mm² on /p/ in "hamper" with complete overlap of oral pressure, nasal pressure, and nasal airflow during the /mp/ segments.

 Listen to Audio 3.3.14.

Audio Case Study 3.3.15

(*Note.* This child is also presented in Video 3.4.9.)

This is an almost 7-year-old female with neurofibromatosis 1 (NF1) (see sidebar) who was referred by her school-based SLP to the cleft palate–craniofacial team because of concerns about hypernasal speech. She does not have a cleft palate.

> Neurofibromatosis 1 (NF1) is an inherited genetic disorder characterized by café au lait spots and growth of tumors along the nerves (called neurofibromas). The tumors can affect the optic nerve and cranial nerves. Individuals can have normal intelligence, and others can have attention-deficit hyperactivity disorder (ADHD) and learning challenges. Low muscle tone, atypical phonation, and hypernasality have been documented. The symptoms vary in severity.

Case History

(*Additional information about this child's medical background is provided in the history for Video 3.4.9*)

Surgical: Tonsillectomy and adenoidectomy (T&A) to relieve obstructive sleep apnea (OSA). This procedure did not alleviate the OSA symptoms. As per parent report, there was no change in this child's speech after the T&A.

Dental: Missing central and lateral incisors

Hearing: An audiological evaluation completed at the time of this assessment showed normal hearing, bilaterally.

Speech Therapy: She was enrolled in Early Intervention until age 3 years, after which she attended a school for children with special needs in an integrated and developmentally appropriate setting until age 5 years. She is in Grade 1, where she receives physical, occupational, and speech therapies.

Studies of Velopharyngeal Function: Pressure-flow studies showed estimated mean areas on /p/ in syllables and "hamper" that exceeded 20 mm^2. Imaging of the velopharyngeal port using multiview videofluoroscopy and videonasoendoscopy showed very little palatal movement and lateral pharyngeal wall movement during phonation, resulting in a large velopharyngeal gap (see videonasoendoscopic assessment in Video 3.4.9).

 Listen to Audio 3.3.15.

Audio Case Study 3.3.16

This is an almost 4-year-old male with repaired left unilateral cleft lip and palate who was internationally adopted at 21 months of age, after lip repair. The palate was unrepaired. He has a history of OME and conductive hearing loss.

Case History

Surgical: Cleft lip was repaired in the country of birth prior to adoption. Palate repair at 22 months after he joined his adoptive family.

Dental: Anterior crossbite

Hearing: An audiological evaluation completed at the time of this assessment showed normal hearing, bilaterally.

Speech Therapy: Started speech therapy through Early Intervention and is currently receiving treatment at school to correct articulation errors.

Listen to Audio 3.3.16.

Audio Case Study 3.3.17

(*Note.* This child is also presented in Video 3.4.11.)

This 6-year-old female was referred to the cleft palate team by her school-based SLP because of hypernasal speech and the presence of a bifid uvula. During her team visit, the surgeon confirmed a diagnosis of submucous cleft palate based on the findings of a notch in the hard palate and partial zone of lucency in the midline.

Case History

Surgical: None to date

Dental: Class I occlusion

Hearing: No history of OME. An audiological evaluation completed at the time of this assessment showed normal hearing, bilaterally.

Speech Therapy: At the time of this visit, she was not receiving speech therapy.

 Listen to Audio 3.3.17.

Audio Case Study 3.3.18

(*Note.* This child is also presented in Video 3.4.16.)

This is a 3.5-year-old male with repaired right unilateral cleft lip and palate who was internationally adopted at 32 months.

Case History

Surgical: The lip was repaired in the country of birth (date unknown) and the palate was repaired at 33 months, 1 month after his adoption. PE tubes inserted at the time of palate repair.

Dental: Class I molar relationship

Hearing: An audiological evaluation completed at the time of this assessment showed a mild conductive hearing loss in the left ear and normal hearing in the right ear.

Speech Therapy: The patient was enrolled in speech therapy after the palate was repaired and was receiving this service at the time of this assessment. The focus of treatment was to achieve correct articulatory placement for oral consonants and eliminate compensatory articulation errors associated with cleft palate.

> ***Listen to Audio 3.3.18.***

Speech Sample (provided to facilitate listening)

- Counting 1 to 10
- Put the baby by the buggy
- Take Teddy to town
- Sissy sees the sky
- Go get the wagon for the girl
- The ship goes in the shallow water
- Jim and Charlie chew gum
- Mama made lemon jam

Audio Case Study 3.3.19

(*Note*. This child's speech was recorded before surgery to correct VPD. You will hear his audio in 3.3.20, one year after surgery.)

This is a 9-year-old male with repaired right unilateral cleft lip and palate. He was internationally adopted at almost 3 years of age.

Case History

Surgical: The cleft lip and palate were repaired in the child's country of birth before his arrival to this country. He underwent maxillary alveolar cleft repair at age 8 years.

Dental: Mixed dentition and Class III malocclusion

Hearing: History is positive for OME treated with PE tubes and fluctuating conductive hearing loss when the OME was present. At the time of this assessment, hearing was within normal limits bilaterally.

Speech Therapy: He has a history of speech therapy and currently receives this service at school to remediate his presenting articulation errors.

 Listen to Audio 3.3.19.

Audio Case Study 3.3.20

(*Note.* This is an audio of the child presented in Audio 3.3.19 one year after surgery to correct VPD. He is now 11 years old.)

Case History

<u>Surgical</u>: At age 10 years, this patient underwent pushback revision palatoplasty with buccal flaps (see sidebar) to correct VPD.

> Pushback revision palatoplasty with buccal flaps is a type of surgical technique to correct VPD. The soft and hard palates are separated and bilateral buccal (cheek) flaps are interposed to lengthen the palate.

<u>Dental</u>: Class III malocclusion and anterior crossbite

<u>Hearing</u>: Within normal limits, bilaterally

<u>Speech Therapy</u>: History of speech therapy to correct articulation errors and continues to receive this service in school

> ### *Listen to Audio 3.3.20.*

■ Section 4. Video Case Studies: Independent Practice

Introduction

This section contains a series of videos of a variety of speakers with and without cleft palate who exhibit speech and resonance disorders. In some cases, the patient's videonasoendoscopic assessment is also shown. Some videos will show speakers pre- and post physical management (surgical, prosthetic). Watch the video and listen to each speaker carefully, noting the features of the communication disorder(s) that are present in each case. We recommend that you use a systems approach to these evaluation practice exercises (see Box 3–2). That is, listen to each sample and evaluate according to the supporting speech systems of resonation, articulation, and phonation. Also consider other parameters such nasal air emission and the presence or absence of facial grimace. We also refer you to Box 3–3 for guiding questions during this process. You are also encouraged to consider recommendations about treatment. Our discussion about each case is presented in Appendix B at the end of this book with which you can compare your findings and recommendations.

Box 3–3. Guiding Questions to Help Direct the Evaluation Process

Assessment Parameters	Questions	Considerations
Resonance	Is there a problem with resonance? Many of our patients with VPI exhibit resonance problems, and the definitions of each are included for review purposes.	A. Hypernasality: perception of excessive nasal resonance during the production of voiced speech sounds, particularly vowels, glides, and liquids. Is resonance WNL or is there hypernasality? What is the perceived degree of hypernasality? Is it mild, moderate, or severe? B. Hyponasality: lack of nasal resonance during the production of nasal consonants and adjacent vowels. Is there a perceived lack of nasal resonance? C. Mixed nasality: components of both hypernasality and hyponasality are perceived in the patient's speech. Are both hyper- and hyponasality present in the patient's speech? If there is a problem, what is the best course of action for the patient? Is there a treatment or treatments that are appropriate for the patient? Is referral to another professional(s) appropriate for this patient? Is the patient being managed for the problem and contact needs to be made with another health care specialist? (See Chapter 5 for Referring to a Cleft Palate Team)

Assessment Parameters	Questions	Considerations
Nasal air emission	Is nasal air emission obligatory due to VPD or fistula, or learned as part of a posterior nasal fricative?	If there is a problem of nasal air emission, categorize it as visible (only on mirror testing), audible, or turbulent. If there is a problem, what is the best course of action for this patient?
Nasal grimace	Is nasal grimacing present during speech?	The speaker with severe VPD may constrict his or her nares during the production of high-pressure oral segments of speech in response to obligatory nasal air emission. Some speakers who use anterior nasal fricatives may also grimace. If there is a problem, what is the best course of action for this patient?
Articulation	Is there an articulation problem? Patients with VPI often show articulation problems.	If articulation problems are present, categorize them according to the classification system presented in the book (refer to Chapter 1). Classify according to the categories of obligatory (adaptive) oral distortions, compensatory (maladaptive), other unusual articulations (i.e., nasal fricatives), developmental, or other coexisting problems.

Assessment Parameters	Questions	Considerations
Articulation *continued*		If there is a problem, what is the best course of action for the patient? Is there a treatment or treatments that are appropriate for the patient? Is referral to another professional(s) appropriate for this patient? Is the patient being managed for the problem and contact needs to be made with another health care specialist?
Phonation	Do you perceive a phonatory problem?	Consider the perceptual parameters of pitch, loudness, and quality. Is the patient's pitch too high, too low, or WNL? Is vocal loudness too high, too low, or WNL? What is the quality of the patient's voice? Is there a vocal quality problem such as hoarseness, harshness, or breathiness? Is voice quality WNL?
		If there is a problem, what is the best course of action for the patient? Is there a treatment or treatments that are appropriate for the patient? Is referral to another professional(s) appropriate for this patient? Is the patient being managed for the problem and contact needs to be made with another health care specialist?

WNL = within normal limits.

Video Case Study 3.4.1

This is a 2-year-old female with repaired complete cleft of the secondary palate.

Case History

Surgical: Palate repair at 12 months. OME treated with PE tubes at the time of palate repair.

Hearing: Recent audiological assessment showed responses to stimuli presented in sound field were within normal limits for at least the better ear.

Speech Therapy: Not enrolled in speech therapy

 Watch Video 3.4.1.

Video Case Study 3.4.2

This is a 6-year-old male with repaired isolated cleft of the secondary palate.

Case History

<u>Surgical</u>: Palate repair at age 10 months. OME treated with PE tubes.

<u>Dental</u>: Mixed dentition. Class II molar relationship on the right, Class I molar relationship on the left.

<u>Hearing</u>: Minimal mild sensorineural hearing loss at 2000 Hz, bilaterally. Normal middle ear function in both ears.

<u>Speech Therapy</u>: History of speech therapy for an articulation disorder.

Watch Video 3.4.2.

Video Case Study 3.4.3

This is a 14-year-old female with repaired left unilateral cleft lip and palate. She was internationally adopted at age 5 years, following lip and palate repair. She first presented to the cleft palate team at age 6. Throughout the years, the family considered this teen's speech to be acceptable. During the most recent team assessment, however, they reported that hypernasality has become more noticeable during conversational speech and that the teachers notice it as well. This teen indicated that she is aware of the nasality and is interested in improving her speech.

This video includes this teen's speech sample and her nasoendoscopic assessment of velopharyngeal function.

Case History

Surgical: Lip and palate repair done in her country of birth. A residual fistula in the hard palate was repaired after she joined her family. Alveolar cleft repair at age 9 years.

Dental: Maxillary expansion was completed prior to alveolar cleft repair. Orthodontic treatment is complete. She currently presents with a Class I occlusal relationship.

Hearing: Within normal limits, bilaterally

Speech Therapy: She has an extensive history of speech therapy that focused on the remediation of compensatory articulation errors including pharyngeal fricatives and affricates. These errors have been corrected. She continues to receive speech therapy twice monthly to monitor articulation. It is worth mentioning that she also presented with palatalized /t/ and /d/ but these were spontaneously eliminated after maxillary expansion.

Studies of Velopharyngeal Function: Videonasoendoscopy was first done to image the velopharyngeal port when the speaker was 10 years old. At that time, findings showed asymmetrical palatal elevation with robust closure noted on the right side and incomplete closure on the left side. The gap was judged to be small, with bubbling emanating from the port. An adenoid pad was present.

Given the family's and clinician's recent concerns about a change in resonance, videonasoendoscopy was repeated. This assessment is presented in the video.

Watch Video 3.4.3.

Video Case Study 3.4.4

This is a 6-year-old male with repaired right unilateral cleft lip and palate.

Case History

<u>Medical</u>: Oral exam showed a short velum with good elevation during phonation and a Passavant's ridge.

<u>Surgical</u>: Lip repair at 3 months of age; palate repair at 9 months of age; secondary Furlow palatoplasty (see sidebar) at approximately 5 years of age.

A Furlow palatoplasty is a type of surgical procedure used for primary cleft palate repair, and it may be used as a secondary treatment for VPD. It corrects malpositioned velar muscles and lengthens the palate.

<u>Dental</u>: Early mixed dentition, reverse overjet, and alveolar cleft

<u>Hearing</u>: Within normal limits, bilaterally

<u>Speech Therapy</u>: Currently enrolled in speech therapy

<u>Pressure-Flow Studies</u>: Findings showed inadequate velopharyngeal closure as suggested by nasal airflow rates exceeding 250 mL/s on /p/ in syllables.

 Watch Video 3.4.4.

Video Case Study 3.4.5

This is an 11-year-old male with repaired bilateral cleft lip and palate. Attendance to the cleft clinic has been irregular.

Case History

<u>Surgical</u>: Lip repair was done at 3 months and palate closure at 12 months. An alveolar bone graft was done at 9 years of age.

<u>Dental</u>: Class III occlusion with a lateral crossbite.

<u>Hearing</u>: At the time of testing, hearing was within normal limits, bilaterally.

<u>Speech Therapy</u>: The patient has a history of speech treatment but is no longer receiving this service.

<u>Studies of Velopharyngeal Function</u>: Pressure-flow studies showed reduced oral pressure in the presence on concomitant nasal air pressure and airflow. Estimates of velopharyngeal orifice opening ranged from 3 to 5 mm^2. Videonasoendoscopy showed a coronal pattern of velopharyngeal movement with a large central gap.

Watch Video 3.4.5.

Video Case Study 3.4.6

(*Note.* This is the same case presented in Audio 3.3.11. In this video, she is seen in before and after surgery to improve speech and resonance).

This is an 18-year-old female with repaired left unilateral cleft lip and palate. She first presented to the cleft palate team at age 7, at which time resonance was judged to be within functional limits. Speech assessments over the course of subsequent team visits suggested gradual changes in resonance. Pressure-flow studies confirmed this change over time. However, the family and patient were reluctant to proceed with surgery to correct VPD until this recent assessment when the patient reported that she was entering college and would like to sound better.

Case History

Surgical: Lip repair at 5 months and palate repair at 12 months. The maxillary alveolar cleft repair is completed. Pushback revision palatoplasty with buccal flaps at 18 years of age to correct VPD.

Dental: Currently in active orthodontics. Class I molar relationship.

Hearing: Mild conductive hearing loss at 4000 to 6000 Hz in the right ear and a moderate to mild conductive hearing loss at the specific frequencies 250, 1000, and 4000 Hz in the left ear.

Speech Therapy: No known history of speech therapy

Studies of Velopharyngeal Function: Pressure-flow studies showed estimated mean areas on /p/ in syllables and "hamper" that exceeded 20 mm^2. Imaging of the velopharyngeal port using both multiview videofluoroscopy and videonasoendoscopy showed incomplete velar closure and minimal lateral pharyngeal wall movement, resulting in a coronal pattern of velopharyngeal closure.

 Watch Video 3.4.6.

Video Case Study 3.4.7

This is an 11-year-old-male who, at age 8, first presented to the cleft palate team due to concerns about hypernasal resonance. He does not have a cleft palate. The mother reported that her son, as a toddler, sounded nasal. Oral examination revealed asymmetrical velar movement during the production of /a/. Videonasoendoscopy confirmed palatal asymmetry. Findings showed robust velopharyngeal closure on the left side and incomplete closure on the right side. Surgery to correct VPD was done when he was 9 years old, after which the mother reported an improvement in resonance. Recently, however, this child requested a speech reevaluation because he perceived an increase in his nasality, and the mother agreed.

Case History

Surgical: Adenoidectomy at 2 years of age with no reported noticeable change in resonance. Two sets of PE tubes to treat OME. Pharyngoplasty with fat graft to posterior pharyngeal wall at age 9.

Dental: Class III occlusion. He is currently wearing a quad helix, an orthodontic appliance used to widen the upper jaw.

Hearing: Within normal limits, bilaterally

Speech Therapy: History of speech therapy from kindergarten through third grade

Listen to his speech during citation and conversation.

Watch Video 3.4.7.

Video Case Study 3.4.8

This is a 15-year-old male with Crouzon syndrome with maxillary hypoplasia (see sidebar). He is scheduled to undergo mandibular advancement and LeFort I osteotomy for maxillary advancement using distraction osteogenesis (MADO) (refer to sidebar under Audio 3.3.1).

> Crouzon syndrome is a genetic disorder characterized by craniosynostosis (premature closure of the cranial sutures), midface hypoplasia, shallow eye orbits, ocular proptosis, and hypertelorism. The maxilla is hypoplastic and retruded, and the mandible, relative to the maxilla, looks prognathic, resulting in a Class III malocclusion.

Case History

<u>Medical</u>: He has a history of obstructive sleep apnea, snoring, and mouth breathing.

<u>Surgical</u>: Cranial vault expansion with fronto-orbital advancement at age 3 years. Tonsillectomy and adenoidectomy at 13 years.

<u>Dental</u>: Skeletal Class III malocclusion. He has undergone orthodontic preparation for surgery. He currently is wearing braces.

<u>Hearing</u>: Within normal limits, bilaterally

 Watch Video 3.4.8.

Video Case Study 3.4.9

(*Note.* This is the same case presented in Audio 3.3.15.)

This 6-year-old female with inherited NF1 was referred to the cleft palate–craniofacial team by her school-based SLP because of concerns about hypernasal speech. She does not have a cleft palate.

This video includes this child's speech sample and her nasoendoscopic assessment of velopharyngeal function. We recognize that the audio signal is reduced.

Case History

Medical: History is also significant for chemotherapy at 21 months for bilateral optic gliomas (she is blind in the right eye), seizure disease, and Moyamoya disease (a rare, progressive blood vessel or vascular disorder in which the carotid artery in the skull becomes blocked or narrowed, reducing blood flow to the brain). She has obstructive sleep apnea (OSA). She does not have a history of ear disease or hearing loss. She does not experience nasal regurgitation.

Surgical: Right parietotemporal craniotomy to treat stenosis arteries associated with Moyamoya disease at 21 months. Tonsillectomy and adenoidectomy done to relieve OSA, but it did not relieve or reduce the symptoms and OSA persists.

Dental: Missing central and lateral incisors

Hearing: At the time of testing, hearing was within normal limits, bilaterally.

Speech Therapy: Received Early Intervention until age 3 years and attended a school for children with special needs in an integrated and developmentally appropriate setting when she was 4 and 5 years old. She is currently a first grader and receives physical, occupational, and speech therapies.

Studies of Velopharyngeal Function: Pressure-flow studies showed estimated mean areas on /p/ in syllables and "hamper" that exceeded 20 mm^2. Imaging of the velopharyngeal port using both multiview videofluoroscopy insert and videonaso-endoccopy showed minimal velar and lateral pharyngeal wall movement during phonation, resulting in a large velopharyngeal gap. The videonasoendoscopy is shown here.

Watch Video 3.4.9. *Note.* In this conversational speech sample, the child is talking about the movie *Frozen*.

Video Case Study 3.4.10

(*Note.* This is the same case presented in Audio 3.2.11.)

This is an 8-year-old female who was referred to the cleft palate team by the school-based SLP because of concerns about nasal resonance. She has low muscle tone and learning challenges.

Case History

Medical: The team surgeon diagnosed a submucous cleft palate on the basis of a bifid uvula, partial zone of lucency in the midline, and a small notch in the posterior hard palate. This child also has a history of OME.

Surgical: None to date

Dental: Open-bite malocclusion associated with a thumbsucking habit

Hearing: Recently received PE tubes to treat otitis media. Before tube insertion, she exhibited a mild bilateral conductive hearing loss. Hearing testing following PE tube insertion was within normal limits, bilaterally.

Speech Therapy: Enrolled in speech therapy

Pressure-Flow Studies: Findings showed nasal air pressure in synchrony with oral pressure during production of the /mp/ sequence in "hamper," which is suggestive of VPD.

Watch Video 3.4.10.

Video Case Study 3.4.11

(*Note*. This case was also presented in Audio 3.3.17.)

This is a 6-year-old female who was referred to the cleft palate team for issues related to resonance. The team surgeon confirmed the diagnosis of submucous cleft palate.

This video includes this child's speech sample and her nasoendoscopic assessment of velopharyngeal function. The nasoendoscopy was performed 2 months after the speech recording and initiation of speech therapy for the remediation of /s/.

Case History

Surgical: None to date

Dental: Class I molar relationship

Hearing: At the time of testing, hearing was within normal limits, bilaterally.

Speech Therapy: At the time of this speech sample, this child had never been enrolled in speech therapy.

 Watch Video 3.4.11.

Video Case Study 3.4.12

(*Note.* This is the same case presented in Audio 3.3.14.)

This is an almost 8-year-old male with repaired bilateral cleft lip and palate who was internationally adopted at 15 months of age. History is significant for OME and associated hearing loss.

Case History

<u>Surgical</u>: Cleft lip was repaired in the country of birth prior to adoption. Palate repair at 17 months after he joined his adoptive family. PE tubes were inserted at the time of palate repair.

<u>Dental</u>: Early mixed dentition. Skeletal Class III. Anterior crossbite and a left crossbite in the canine and first molar region. Bilateral maxillary alveolar clefts with oronasal fistulas are present, but the child is not yet ready for maxillary expansion in preparation for alveolar cleft repair.

<u>Hearing</u>: At the time of testing, he exhibited a mild low-frequency conductive hearing loss, bilaterally.

<u>Speech Therapy</u>: This child started speech therapy as part of an Early Intervention program and continued when he entered school. He is currently receiving treatment at school and also through a hospital-based program to correct articulation errors associated with the cleft.

<u>Pressure-Flow Studies</u>: Findings showed estimated VP areas exceeding that of 20 mm^2 on /p/ in "hamper" with complete overlap of oral pressure, nasal pressure, and nasal airflow during /mp/ segments. These findings are consistent with inadequate VP closure.

Watch Video 3.4.12.

Video Case Study 3.4.13

This is an almost 7-year-old male with a repaired submucous cleft palate and history of OME. He first presented to the cleft palate team at 4 years old upon the referral of the otolaryngologist. This diagnosis of submucous cleft palate was based on the presence of a bifid uvula, translucent zone in the midline of the soft palate, and a notch in the posterior hard palate.

Case History

<u>Surgical</u>: Palate repair at 5 years. OME treated with PE tubes at time of palate repair.

<u>Dental</u>: Class II occlusion

<u>Hearing</u>: At the time of testing, hearing was within normal limits, bilaterally.

<u>Speech Therapy</u>: Enrolled for the first time in speech therapy at age 4 years prior to team visit and continues to receive these services to correct articulation errors.

 Watch Video 3.4.13.

Video Case Study 3.4.14

This is a 3-year-old male with repaired left unilateral cleft lip and palate.

Case History

Surgical: Lip repair at 3 months and palate at 12 months. OME treated with PE tubes at the time of palate repair.

Dental: Class III and posterior crossbite. Missing left lateral incisor. Maxillary alveolar cleft repair will be done during the mixed stage of dentition between 7 and 10 years.

Hearing: At the time of testing, this child exhibited a mild-moderate conductive hearing loss in speech frequency range in at least one ear and Type B tympanometric configurations bilaterally, suggestive of middle ear pathology. He is scheduled to have the PE tubes replaced.

Speech Therapy: Enrolled in speech therapy

> ### *Watch Video 3.4.14.*

Note. This child is producing words from the Arizona Articulation Proficiency Scale-2. A list of the words he is producing is provided to facilitate your understanding (few are completely unintelligible as shown by ??). He also produces a few spontaneous comments during the test.

Words: horse, nine, tree, cup, bath, comb, TV, cook, stove, ladder, ball, yellow, vanilla, bird, fork, ??, car, ear, ring, trees, ??, green, watch, zipper, nose, nest, carrot, books, cake, wagon

Video Case Study 3.4.15

(*Note*. This child was 3.5 years old when he was presented in Audio 3.2.19. In this video, he is school aged.)

This is a 5-year-old male with repaired left unilateral cleft lip and palate who was internationally adopted at age 3. He first presented to the cleft palate team at age 3.5 years.

This video includes this child's speech sample and naso-endoscopic assessment of velopharyngeal function.

Case History

Surgical: Lip and palate repair completed by 1 year in birth country prior to adoption. OME treated with PE tubes.

Dental: Class I occlusion. Maxillary alveolar cleft with a very narrow oronasal fistula high in the vestibule.

Hearing: Responses to stimuli presented in sound field were within normal limits for at least the better ear. Otoscopy revealed tympanic membrane perforation in the right ear and PE tube in the left ear.

Speech Therapy: Enrolled in speech therapy to improve articulation.

Studies of Velopharyngeal Function: Pressure-flow testing showed estimated velopharyngeal areas of 20.0 mm^2 on "hamper." There was complete overlap of oral pressure, nasal pressure, and nasal airflow during /-mp/ segments. In other words, the oral-nasal coupling was so complete that this child was unable to aerodynamically distinguish the /m/ from the /p/ segments in words. Estimated areas on /p/ in /papapa/ and /pipipi/ also exceeded 20 mm^2. Multiview videofluoroscopy showed a moderately sized velopharyngeal gap characterized by a coronal closure pattern.

 Watch Video 3.4.15.

Video Case Study 3.4.16

(*Note.* This is the same child presented in Audio 3.3.18.)

This is a child with a repaired right unilateral cleft lip and palate who was internationally adopted at 32 months. In the first segment of this video, is 3.5 years old. In the second segment, he is 14 years old.

Case History

Surgical: Lip repair in this child's country of birth (date unknown). The palate was repaired at 33 months, 1 month after his arrival to this country. At age 6, he underwent sphincter pharyngoplasty to correct VPD and alveolar cleft repair at 9 years. PE tubes to treat OME were done at the time of palate repair with repeated sets of PE tubes several times thereafter during elementary school years. Maxillary advancement will be done when he has reached skeletal maturity and completed facial growth.

Dental: Class I molar relationship at age 3.5 years. By 14 years of age, he developed a skeletal Class III malocclusion associated with maxillary hypoplasia.

Hearing: At the time of testing at 3.5 years of age, this child exhibited a mild conductive hearing loss in the left ear and normal hearing in the right ear. During his recent audiological testing at age 14, hearing was within normal limits, bilaterally.

Speech Therapy: Speech therapy was initiated after palate repair. The focus of treatment was to achieve correct articulatory placement for oral consonants and eliminate compensatory errors associated with cleft palate. Articulation errors were all corrected but hypernasal speech persisted. Videonasoendoscopy confirmed the presence of a velopharyngeal gap for which surgery to correct VPD was recommended. He did not receive speech therapy after surgery to correct VPD.

Note. In the first segment, this child is producing words from the Arizona Articulation Proficiency Scale-2. A list of the words he is producing is provided to facilitate your understanding (see below). He also produces a small conversational speech sample.

<u>Words</u>: telephone, cup, knife, ball, ring, shovel, banana, zipper (first try), zipper (second try with imitation), scissors, vacuum, watch, airplane, counting 1 to 5, 7.

Watch Video 3.4.16.

Video Case Study 3.4.17

(*Note.* Before and after insertion of speech appliance to correct VPD.)

This is a 10-year-old female with Pierre Robin sequence and a repaired cleft of the soft palate. She presented with hypernasal speech and compensatory speech sound errors. Parents were not interested in a surgical option but wanted a prosthesis fabricated for the patient, which was done. In the first segment of the video, you will hear this child's speech without the palatal appliance. In the following segment, you will have the opportunity to hear her speech while she wears the speech appliance.

Case History

Surgical: The palatal defect was repaired at 12 months and a fistula developed, which was later surgically closed.

Dental: Dentition is within normal limits.

Hearing: At the time of testing, hearing was within normal limits, bilaterally.

Speech Therapy: She presented with hypernasality and compensatory speech sound errors. She did receive treatment for the compensatory errors.

Studies of Velopharyngeal Function: Pressure-flow studies showed reduced oral pressure in the presence of concomitant nasal air pressure and airflow. Videonasoendoscopy showed a coronal pattern of velopharyngeal movement without complete closure.

Watch Video 3.4.17.

Video Case Study 3.4.18

(*Note.* Before and after surgery to correct VPD.)

This is an 8.5-year-old male with repaired isolated cleft of the secondary palate who first presented to the cleft palate team at age 3 years. Speech assessments over the course of subsequent team visits suggested gradual changes in resonance and confirmed using pressure-flow studies. In this video, you will have the opportunity to follow this child through the course of his treatment. In Part 1, you will hear his speech when he is 5 years old and receiving speech therapy. In Part 2, he is 8 years old. You will first hear a sample of his speech followed by his nasoendoscopic assessment of VP function. In Part 3, you will hear his speech 9 weeks after surgery to correct VPD.

Case History

Surgical: Palate repair at 9 months of age. PE tubes to treat OME at the time of palate repair. Pushback revision palatoplasty with buccal flaps (see sidebar 3.3.20) at age 8.5 years to correct VPD.

Dental: Class I molar relationship; slight crossbite on left side

Hearing: At the time of testing, hearing was within normal limits, bilaterally.

Speech Therapy: He has a history of speech therapy to correct articulation errors. At age 5 years, he was enrolled in speech therapy to improve articulation for /s, z, ʃ, /tʃ/ and continued to receive this service throughout the course of his treatment.

Preoperative Studies of Velopharyngeal Function: Pressure-flow testing indicated incomplete (or marginal) velopharyngeal closure as evidenced by nasal airflow exceeding 106 mL/s during /pi/. Multiview videofluoroscopy showed incomplete velar closure and minimal lateral pharyngeal wall movement resulting in a coronal pattern of velopharyngeal closure.

Postoperative Studies of Velopharyngeal Function at 9 Weeks: Pressure-flow testing showed a change in velopharyngeal function as evident by a reduction in nasal airflow rates that ranged from 15 to 24 mL/s during /pi/.

Watch Video 3.4.18.

Video Case Study 3.4.19

(*Note.* Before and after surgery to improve velopharyngeal function.)

This final video is that of a 10-year-old female with congenital ectodermal dysplasia, as part of Bartsocas Papas syndrome (BPS) (see sidebar) and bilateral cleft lip and palate. She is shown during her course of treatment for VPD. In the first segment of the video, she is 5 years old, during which time she was enrolled in speech. In the second segment, she is 10 years old and 3 months postsurgery to correct VPD.

Bartsocas Papas syndrome (BPS) is a rare inherited syndrome that includes facial clefts and additional ectodermal dysplasia anomalies (i.e., absent/ sparse hair, eyebrows, lashes, nails).

Case History

Medical: Born at 34 weeks' gestation. Very protrusive premaxilla deviated to the left side and underdeveloped soft palate musculature. Recurrent episodes of OME. History of OSA.

Surgical:
- 8 weeks: Presurgical palatal appliance (see sidebar)
- 4 months: Appliance was removed and a bilateral lip adhesion was done.
- 7 months: Definitive lip repair at 7 months
- 11 months: Palate repair and PE tubes at the time of palate repair to manage OME (note: PE tubes were replaced three times, thereafter)
- 4 years: Pushback revision palatoplasty with buccal flaps to correct VPD
- 8 years: Maxillary alveolar cleft repair
- 9.9 years: VPD persisted after the pushback revision procedure (see sidebar 3.3.20). After this, the child was

reevaluated for OSA and considered to no longer be at risk for the condition, and a sphincter pharyngoplasty was done to correct VPD.

> The presurgical palatal appliance is mainly used to retract and align the protruded and deviated pre-maxilla and to facilitate initial lip repair

Dental: Class III with posterior crossbite

Hearing: At the time of testing, hearing within normal limits, bilaterally.

Speech Therapy: Early history of speech therapy to correct compensatory articulation errors associated with VPD

Studies of Velopharyngeal Function: Imaging of the velo-pharyngeal port using both multiview videofluoroscopy and videonasoendoscopy was done at age 9. Findings showed incomplete velar closure and minimal lateral pharyngeal wall movement, resulting in a coronal pattern of velopharyngeal closure. Instrumental findings confirmed the presence of VPD and a sphincter pharyngoplasty was recommended.

Watch Video 3.4.19.

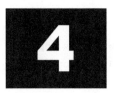

4

Treatment

Introduction

For several of the cases in Chapter 3, we documented via video recordings the interactive effect of surgical intervention and speech therapy. Although surgery can and does improve VPD in most cases, the articulation errors present before surgery may continue to persist afterwards. These errors warranted treatment that was delivered by SLPs in the community who were guided by specific recommendations of the respective team SLPs. In that chapter, we also presented cases for which speech treatment alone was considered to be the most appropriate recommendation.

Treatment for patients with cleft palate targets compensatory (maladaptive), other unusual articulations, and any coexisting disorders that are amenable to speech-language treatment. For instance, the patient may also present with a phonatory disorder, and a treatment program for the disorder would be implemented as part of an overall treatment plan. Generally, treatment directed to VPD in order to modify hypernasality is not advisable, since there is substantial literature that has not supported different behavioral treatments for improving VPD (Lof & Ruscello, 2013; Ruscello, 2004; Tomes, Kuehn, & Peterson-Falzone, 2004).

This chapter describes treatment strategies to correct speech errors that are amenable to therapy. Initially, general treatment concepts will be discussed as a basis for understanding and using recommended treatment methods and techniques. This will be followed by different treatment methods and techniques that are part of the literature and have been used with reported supporting evidence. Finally, a teaching technology will also be discussed for use in treatment. Readers should be aware of the fact that the evidence base for different treatments is lacking. There is some limited evidence from randomized studies, cohort studies, case studies, descriptive studies, and expert opinion (Bessell et al., 2013; Vallino-Napoli, 2011). Where applicable, the evidence level will be cited for the reader using the criteria presented by Justice and Fey (2004).

■ Approach to Treatment

One of the issues that has been debated in the literature is the basis for the speech errors (compensatory and other unusual articulations) produced by patients with cleft palate. Are they phonetic errors or phonemic errors? Some SLPs propose that the sound system errors of patients with VPD are phonologically based (Chapman, 1993; Pamplona & Ysunza, 1999); however, there is a physiological cause that underlies many of the errors. For example, Golding-Kushner (2001) explains that a glottal stop is a physiologically based compensatory error, not a phonologically based error. This would mean that there is a change in the patient's motor output, rather than an error at the phonologic level. The assumption is that the patient has developed the phonological representations of the phonemes. That is, the patient has formed the appropriate acoustic-phonetic representations for various stored lexical items and developed linkages with semantic representations and motor planning (Rvachew & Brosseau-Lapre, 2018). In our case, it is the structural problem that prevents the patient from processing the appropriate phonological representations for production. That is, the patient has the appropriate representations in storage and is capable of planning the appropriate motor commands, but execution is problematic due to a structural deficit. Trost-Cardamone and Bernthal (1993) write,

> Although we do not know the extent to which early oral structural deviations associated with cleft palate interfere with acquisition of underlying phonological representations, the child with compensatory substitutions has problems with place features at the surface level. For this reason, the clinician should focus instruction on teaching place contrasts within the vocal tract, for the stops, fricatives, and affricates. (p. 330)

We agree with Trost-Cardamone and Bernthal and discuss treatment from that perspective, but note that some patients may indeed exhibit phonemic errors in addition to phonetic-based compensatory and other unusual articulation errors. The presence of phonemic positional constraints and/or inventory constraints in the patient's phonology would be suggestive of a phonological component to the speech sound disorder. As a result, such errors would be subject to phonemic-based treatment concepts.

■ General Treatment Concepts

1. Patients with cleft palate are typically followed by a craniofacial team for tertiary care and receive primary and secondary care from community-based resources. Grames (2004) writes that in the case of SLP services, a patient has been followed from birth, and recommendations for speech treatment are made by the team. SLPs should be aware of the fact that there are a number of innovative

collaborative models, and selection of the most appropriate will vary as a function of the patient, caregivers, and SLPs involved in the care of the patient (Grames & Stahl, 2017). In some cases, there can be obstacles to effective collaboration, because the SLP who carries out the treatment does not have extensive experience with such patients, and the care philosophies underlying the two organizations differ. The most important factors in collaboration are keeping an open line of communication and shared control of the patient. If there are any problems with treatment recommendations, the patient's SLP should consult with the team SLP. It may also be beneficial to accompany the patient on a visit to the cleft palate team.

2. Surgery for cleft lip and palate generally happens prior to 18 months of age. In most cases, it has been done during the first year of life. Estimates suggest that approximately 70% to 75% of patients undergoing palatal repair develop normal speech (Morris, 1992; Zajac & Vallino, 2017).

3. In some patients, VPD may persist after initial palatal repair. These patients will require a secondary surgery such as, but not limited to, a pharyngeal flap, sphincter pharyngoplasty, or palatal revision with buccal flap, or be fitted with a speech appliance in order to improve velopharyngeal function. If compensatory or other unusual articulation (i.e., nasal fricatives) errors are present in the patient's speech, treatment should not be delayed until surgery or prosthetic intervention. The delivery of treatment will differ in terms of the patient's chronological age and level of development (Trost-Cardamone, 2013).

4. Compensatory and maladaptive errors should be targeted for treatment. Compensatory speech sound errors include glottal stops, pharyngeal fricatives, pharyngeal affricates, and pharyngeal stops (Trost-Cardamone, 2013). Other unusual articulation include anterior and posterior nasal fricatives (see Chapter 1). Developmental errors may or may not be targets for treatment depending on the chronological age of the patient. Generally, obligatory or adaptive errors are not targets for treatment, since the errors are due to a

structural problem. Referral is frequently necessary to other disciplines such as dental and/or medical specialists.

5. Some studies have demonstrated that the correction of compensatory errors has a positive influence on velopharyngeal movement (Henningsson & Isberg, 1986). That is, modifying compensatory errors can facilitate velopharyngeal movement toward closure for speech, but hypernasality and nasal emission may remain to some degree (Trost-Cardamone, 2013). Hypernasality is a resonance disorder and nasal emission is an aerodynamic event, and both are obligatory due to VPD.

6. Parent involvement is an important component of treatment. Parents who show a willingness to participate in their child's treatment should be recruited to conduct home practice sessions (Scherer, 2017).

7. Patients receiving speech sound treatment and undergoing secondary surgical repair may recommence treatment following clearance by their doctor. It is not necessary to postpone treatment for an extended time (Golding-Kushner, 2001).

8. The majority of patients with cleft palate do not have an orofacial muscle weakness but exhibit compensatory, obligatory (adaptive) oral distortions, and other unusual errors (i.e., nasal fricatives). Nonspeech oral motor treatment techniques such as blowing, sucking, or specific resistance exercises to improve lip or tongue strength are not appropriate (McCauley, Strand, Lof, Schooling, & Frymark, 2009).

9. Studies designed to influence velopharyngeal function through nonspeech oral motor treatments, thus improving resonance balance, have not been successful (Tomes, Kuehn, & Peterson-Falzone, 2004). The evidence does not support the application of nonspeech oral motor exercises (NSOMEs) such as blowing, muscle strengthening, and oral/nasal awareness for patients with cleft palate who have VPD and associated speech production errors (Glaze, 2009; Lof & Ruscello, 2013; Ruscello, 2004). The exercises used during NSOMEs are not relevant to speech movement (Lof & Ruscello, 2013). They are NOT effective as treatment approaches and inappropriate to use in therapy.

10. Patients with cleft palate are vulnerable for middle ear infections and fluctuating hearing loss. The SLP needs to be aware of this problem and assist the patients' parents, teachers, and other caregivers to facilitate appropriate medical, audiological, and educational services.
11. Patients with cleft palate as a group are at risk for language delays (McWilliams, Morris, & Shelton, 1984, 1990; Peterson-Falzone et al., 2010). Initial evaluation and periodic monitoring should be conducted during the preschool years. Language treatment should be initiated if a delay is identified.

■ Treating Toddlers With Cleft Palate

There is evidence to show that some toddlers with cleft palate have limited vocabularies, have restricted sound inventories, and develop compensatory speech sound errors (Scherer, D'Antonio, & McGahey, 2008). It is then logical to provide intervention services as soon as possible to minimize communication delays and development of compensatory errors. Hardin-Jones, Chapman, and Scherer (2006) stress the fact that early intervention should center on increasing speech sound inventories, particularly pressure sounds such as plosives and expanding the patient's vocabulary. There is research evidence at the level of demonstrated effectiveness to support early intervention for patients with cleft palate (Justice & Fey, 2004). That is, the existing evidence does demonstrate that intervention by parents for toddlers with cleft palate can be effective, but such evidence is not at the highest level of experimental control such as a randomized control trial. The following information was adapted from the work of Scherer and her associates (2007, 2008, 2017) and can be used with parents as the primary providers of intervention in a patient-oriented approach to treatment. The treatment is provided by the patient's parents, who are trained by the SLP to carry out the intervention program. Please see Table 4–1 for the components of the program.

Initially, the SLP will need to collect assessment data to establish the patient's speech sound inventory, vocabulary,

Table 4–1. The Components of a Patient-Oriented Home Treatment Program

Component	Program Description
1. Introductory Component	Parents are presented with written and verbal descriptions of speech and language development. They are informed of the potential for communication delays and the use of compensatory errors, particularly glottal stops and maladaptive errors. The class of stop sounds is discussed as a potential target.
2. Parent Training Component	Parents are asked to work with their child at least 5 days per week for 15 to 20 minutes each day. Parents are presented with a listing of books and toys that are to be used with their child. The vocabulary highlights the stop speech sounds. Initially, parents are instructed to present the book(s) and read or discuss the stories with their child. Parents can vary using the book(s), the toys, and also including some of the child's toys. Parents are instructed to make eye contact and position themselves at the level of the child. Stimulation techniques are demonstrated for the parents and then they are observed using the techniques with their child.
3. Implementing Parent Intervention	After a few days of exposure to the book(s), the parent can determine if the child is more interested in the books or the toys. Parents can then use the materials that the child prefers. The following stimulation techniques are used by the parents. **1. Focused stimulation**—is one of the primary techniques that is utilized. It is used to present the target vocabulary with the plosive sounds in the prevocalic word position. During a treatment session, many exemplars are presented in context, so that the child is exposed to numerous models of the target words. Parents are instructed to prolong the first sound (plosive sound) of the word. The parent should say /phhhit/ in a normal loudness level. Facilitating strategies used include: **Repetition**—the parent repeats a word or word approximation that the child has just said, so that the child receives an adult model of the word and verification that the parent was listening.

continues

Table 4–1. *continued*

Component	Program Description
3. **Implementing** **Parent** **Intervention** *continued*	**Interpretation**—the parent can incorporate a word that the child has just said in a sentence. Instruct the parent to be sure of the word that the child said, before it is used in a simple sentence. **Modeling**—the parent talks about what the child is doing. It is a good time to introduce some of the featured vocabulary, when describing the child's actions. **Expansion**—this technique expands upon what the child says. If the child says a word, the parent expands and uses it in a simple sentence. The idea is to add more information about what the child is saying. **2. Enhanced milieu training (EMT) and enhanced milieu training with phonological emphasis (EMT/PE)**—constitute the other primary teaching strategies that are designed to facilitate both sound production and vocabulary development. Additional strategies include: **Responsive interaction**—the parent responds to the child's communicative and nonverbal interactional attempts. **Environment**—parent changes the environment to stimulate interaction. **Other components**—a variety of interactive strategies such as time delay with interactions and others like questioning, expansion, modeling, and speech recasting are all employed to simulate vocabulary development and production of pressure sounds, particularly stops.
4. **SLP Roles in** **Administering** **the Home** **Program**	**Baseline**—collecting initial performance data on the child's speech and language skills. **Materials**—preparing and developing materials to be used in the parent/child dyads. **Training**—training the parent to administer the program. **Contract**—develop a contract in writing concerning the roles and responsibilities of the parent and SLP. **Monitoring**—periodically assessing the child's progress, modifying the parent program if necessary, and consulting with the family when needed.

and overall expressive/receptive language skills. If the patient exhibits a restricted sound inventory, limited vocabulary, and compensatory errors, the parent/patient program is a viable choice, provided that the parents are willing to carry out the program. Parents must be committed to the program, which means that the SLP should clearly explain what is expected of them. If the parent is willing, the SLP should negotiate a contract that summarizes what is to be done and how it is to be done. If the parent agrees to the conditions of the contract, both parties sign it. The introductory component of the program is one of education that involves discussion, the provision of reading materials, and selecting appropriate books and toys. The different teaching techniques that are used to facilitate pressure sound production, language vocabulary stimulation, and expansion are focused stimulation, enhanced milieu training (EMT), and enhanced milieu training with phonological emphasis (EMT/PE). The techniques summarized in Table 4–1 are demonstrated and then practiced by the parents. This is followed by the parent-administered treatment and careful monitoring by the SLP to ensure that the treatment sessions are being conducted correctly.

Scherer and her associates discussed some of the concerns that parents expressed during the treatment period, and the concerns are summarized herein. One concern was that some of the patients did not respond initially to the program. The stimulation techniques did not immediately result in increased verbal output. Parents were instructed to continue with the program and use the stimulation techniques such as focused stimulation and modeling, because some patients take time to respond in the treatment paradigm. They were also instructed to minimize the use of questions with their child. Some parents were concerned about the length of the treatment sessions, and they were told to keep the sessions at 10 to 15 minutes and encourage their child to interact and enjoy the treatment sessions. After a period of transition, the patients became responsive to the different stimulation techniques. Others indicated that their children did not want to end the sessions. The authors instructed the parents to keep the sessions at the expected time period and end them with a cleanup period. This served as a signal that the session was over. In some cases, parents reported that their children's productions of target sounds resulted in audible nasal emission. Parents were told that their children were going through a time period of starting to use the muscles of the palate. Further assessment would be needed as the patient grows older to determine if velopharyngeal closure for speech is achieved. We would agree and also add that the parent "play a game" with the patient by occluding the nostrils and then having the patient do the same for some word productions. This helps the patient impound air and develop adequate oral air pressure for sounds such as the stops.

Supplemental Treatment Techniques to Provide Feedback

When engaging in direct treatment activities, the SLP needs to be cognizant of the fact that many patients with cleft palate may experience problems in achieving the correct placement of target sounds. Compensatory (maladaptive) errors may be very ingrained and may not respond to imitative models alone. Even with therapy to correct those sounds, stimulation needs to be provided, as demonstrated in this example (see video 4.1).

Watch Video 4.1.

Consequently, it may be necessary to provide the patient with additional types of performance feedback or assistance during treatment (Peterson-Falzone, Trost-Cardamone, Karnell, & Hardin-Jones, 2017). The techniques do not have a significant evidence base but rather are based primarily on case studies and the opinion of experts (Justice & Fey, 2004). Some examples of providing additional performance feedback or assistance include the following:

1. A mirror to observe articulatory placements can be helpful to augment the patient's auditory monitoring, especially during the beginning stages of speech sound

acquisition (Trost-Cardamone, 1990a). Diagrams of the articulators showing specific sound placements can also be used to achieve correct sound placements.

2. Digital occlusion of the nostrils is a technique that can assist the patient in impounding oral air pressure for speech production. It will prevent unwanted nasal emission. This method is also known as the cul-de-sac technique. Kummer (20014) indicated that additional tactile feedback is available to the patient, if she or he occludes the nostrils. A nasal clip can also be used to occlude the nostrils.

3. Using whisper in speech can serve as a strategy for minimizing glottal articulations. This can especially be helpful for young patients when used in a play-type situation. Physiologically, the vocal folds approximate and the arytenoids are rotated marginally in but are separated posteriorly, creating an enlarged space in the cartilaginous larynx. Air passing through the opening creates a turbulent noise source. Whisper serves as a starting point for breaking up the glottal articulations and can gradually be phased out of treatment.

4. The use of auditory self-monitoring is a very important skill to teach patients enrolled in treatment (Ruscello, 2008a). When they are taught correct placement for a sound or sounds, they need to be instructed to "listen to their speech and use the sounds made in the mouth by their lips and tongue." They can also be involved in the judgment accuracy of their productions during treatment by having them assess periodically practice items.

5. An additional method of providing auditory focus during treatment is the use of a listening tube. This consists of a small piece of plastic tubing that can be purchased at a home improvement store. The tubing is placed at the lips or nose and positioned near the patient's auditory canal.

6. The Scape device (Pro-Ed, Inc.) can be used for visual feedback of nasal airflow during therapy and at home during practice. The See Scape consists of a nasal olive and flexible tube attached to a rigid cylinder with a float inside. The device is intended to provide visual feedback of nasal airflow by placing the olive in one of the nostrils. Of note, the See Scape can also be used to provide visual

feedback of oral airflow by holding the olive in or near the mouth. This is a typical use of the device to establish oral fricatives when nasal fricatives are present.

7. There is also sophisticated equipment that can be employed for feedback purposes, such as pressure/flow equipment and endoscopy (see Chapter 1). However, many SLPs do not have access to such equipment, because they do not have substantial numbers of patients with cleft palate on their caseloads. Therefore, the previous techniques may provide some inexpensive options for the SLP.

■ Treating the Speech Sound Disorders of Older Patients

Since 1969, a number of studies have examined the effectiveness of direct speech sound treatment for persons with cleft palate (Bessell et al., 2013, Peterson-Falzone et al., 2010). The results indicate that speech sound treatment does result in positive changes for patients with velopharyngeal closure and those who present with VPD. However, the research is limited in scope and experimental control. As a result, the evidence base is limited and would be termed by Justice and Fey (2004) as fair evidence for the support of treatment in this clinical population. This part of treatment will deal with the progression of speech sounds to be introduced in treatment, some techniques for establishing correct oral placements of those sounds, and a teaching technology to be used for this type of phonetic teaching.

Treating Speech Sound Errors

Some researchers such as Golding-Kushner (2001) and Trost-Cardamone (2013) have recommended a specific progression when introducing speech sounds. For example, Golding-Kushner recommends the first speech sound to be introduced is /h/. Following acquisition of /h/, speech sounds are presented in an anterior to posterior point of articulation. Golding-Kushner indicates that the order can be modified if a particular sound or group of sounds is stimulable, or the patient has acquired some pressure sounds and is using them correctly. For instance, Golding-Kushner recommends that bilabials (/m, p, b/) be presented prior to introducing alveolars (/t, d, n/); however, if alveolar sounds are found to be stimulable, the SLP may target them initially. The recommended progression of speech sounds is illustrated in Table 4–2.

Laryngeal

The basis for introducing /h/ initially is that the patient is producing a speech sound that is not physiologically congruent with the production of a glottal stop. The acquisition of /h/ and incorporating it in a core of syllables and then progressing to words is important in the remediation of compensatory errors. Typically, a patient is able to imitate stimuli produced by the SLP. The model can be prolonged to approximate a whisper-type production. When correct target production is achieved, the speech sound is integrated into different word positions (pre-, post-, and intervocalic positions) and levels of practice

Table 4–2. Recommended Progression of Speech Sounds According to Place of Articulation

Place of Articulation	*Phonemes*
Laryngeal place	/h/
Bilabial place	/m, p, b/
Labiodental place	/f, v/
Linguadental place	/θ, ð/
Alveolar place	/n, t, d/ /s, z/
Velar place	/ŋ, g, k/
Palatal place	/ʃ, ʒ/ /tʃ, dʒ/

such as syllables, words, phrases, and sentences. For example, the SLP may initially target /h/ in the prevocalic position of syllables. When the patient achieves the designated response accuracy criterion, practice may shift to a different word position or level of practice material such as phrases, sentences, and conversation. Note that the /h/ speech sound occurs in the pre- and intervocalic word positions.

In addition to minimizing the glottal stop articulations, mastery of /h/ enables the SLP to use /h/ as a coarticulating sound (Trost-Cardamone, 2013). For example, the /h/ can be sustained as an initiating sound in the production of the stop /p/. A teaching sequence such as /hhhhhhpuhh/ could be used to minimize a glottal stop production for /p/, when introducing that sound as a target. It is also recommended that imagery be used to create a contrast between the misarticulation and the target sound (Peterson-Falzone et al., 2017). For example, the SLP may label a glottal stop production as a "coughing sound" and the target sound as a "popping sound that is made with the lips." This is designed to help the patient develop a percept of the intended target and help break up the posterior articulation pattern. In the early stages of treatment, correct productions and errors are noted by the SLP, and appropriate knowledge of results is given to the patient. For example, "No you made the coughing sound. I need you to make the /p/ popping sound!"

Bilabials and Labiodentals

After acquiring correct placement and use of /h/, treatment is directed to the bilabials and labiodentals. The first group of sounds are the bilabials /m, p, b/. Most patients with cleft palate can produce nasals such as /m/; however, if it is not part of the patient's sound inventory, it needs to be taught. Golding-Kushner recommends that the patient be instructed to close the lips and hum a song. This facilitating technique will often result in the correct articulation of /m/. The other bilabials are the plosive cognates /p, b/. These sounds are pressure sounds and require the generation of satisfactory intraoral air pressure for their production. A glottal stop substitution is frequently used in place of the bilabial productions. Golding-

Kushner (2001) suggests that the SLP begin with the voiceless /p/. Instruct the patient to prolong /h/ and then close and open the lips to produce the /p/ sound. With some patients, occluding the nostrils is necessary to prevent air from passing through the nose. Kummer (2014) recommends that the patient be trained to whisper the /p/, including the adjacent vowel, since whispering will prevent vocal fold adduction. Correct production of the cognate /b/ may be elicited by telling the patient to "make the sound like /p/ but turn on your voice," or instruct the patient to articulate an /m/ and then occlude the nostrils to produce correctly /b/ (Trost-Cardamone, 2013). Once place of articulation is achieved, the target sound is then incorporated into different contextual levels of practice.

The SLP generally conceptualizes phonetic practice in terms of linguistic complexity such as a hierarchy that includes syllables, words, phrases, sentences, and spontaneous conversation. The patient practices at different levels and progresses to spontaneous usage of a target or targets. In addition to this generally accepted practice, Dobbelsteyn et al. (2014) presented a practice program that is carried out by parents and known as corrective babbling (CB). It consists of nonsense syllables with the target sound in the prevocalic position with syllable structure including simple and complex syllable shapes. The rationale is to practice the targets in syllables that are devoid of meaning, so that the patient engages in extensive phonetic practice. The published evidence for this treatment would be judged as insufficient at this time due to the limited amount and type of empirical scrutiny that has taken place to date. However, it is a practice paradigm that the SLP might want to consider as an adjunct to treatment, since it also involves the parents and adds a different type of practice response from the patient.

The labiodental fricatives /f, v/ are the next set of sounds to be targeted. In some cases, patients will substitute a pharyngeal fricative for these speech sounds. The patient is directed to prolong the /h/ and then bring the lower lip and upper teeth together to produce the target sound. Golding-Kushner (2001) advises against telling the patient to "bite the lip," as this may cause the patient to develop a restricted constriction of the lip and teeth. When initially producing the sound, the

SLP needs to occlude the patient's nostrils with digital occlusion, because nasal airflow is often directed through the nose. When the patient can direct the airstream orally with the correct point of articulation, digital occlusion may be eliminated. The voiced cognate /v/ is taught by instructing the patient to use the voice when making the sound. Verbal imagery cues such as "buzz like a bee" or "make a humming sound" can be used to assist with voicing. Initial occlusion of the nostrils is also used with the voiced cognate /v/ if needed.

Linguadentals and Alveolars

The next groups of sounds are those produced at the linguadental and alveolar points of articulation and are the first lingual sounds to be introduced. The fricative cognates /θ, ð/ are visible sounds and taught in the same way as the labiodental fricatives /f, v/. The difference is that the placement cues will differ as a function of place of articulation. The patient is told to "place the tongue tip between the teeth and make air come out your mouth." Occluding the nostrils or the use of other feedback techniques may need to be used during the initial teaching of the target sounds, so that the patients can develop a pressure head, requisite to correct sound production. Researchers indicate that /θ, ð/ may serve as facilitating agents for acquiring production of the fricative pair /s, z/; consequently, appropriate placement is important (Golding-Kushner, 2001; Trost-Cardamone, 2013).

The alveolars /n, t, d/ are then presented if the patient does not produce the sounds correctly. The nasal /n/ is taught first. The patient is given the verbal cue "open your mouth a little and touch your tongue behind your upper teeth. Once you touch, you need to let your tongue go." The patient should also be told that /n/ is like /m/, so there will be "some sound coming from the nose." The plosives /t, d/ are taught after the /n/ speech sound. Golding-Kushner (2001) suggests that the sound elicitation technique used for /p, b/ also be employed for /t, d/ since they have the same manner of articulation. The patient is instructed to prolong the /h/ and alternately touch and release the tongue tip as it creates a constriction with the alveolar ridge. This elicitation technique can be modeled for the patient, so that she or he is provided with the appropriate auditory and visual information requisite to production (/hhh-hhhhtuh/). Peterson-Falzone et al. (2017) caution that in some cases, patients produce compensatory errors as coproductions with the target place of articulation. The patient might produce an alveolar /t/ simultaneously with a glottal stop. The SLP must be alert to these error types as they may be difficult to perceive through auditory means.

The alveolar fricatives /s, z/ are often very difficult for patients with cleft palate to produce, and initial treatment should be carried out with the nostrils occluded. Riski (2003) has developed some teaching strategies for eliciting correct production of /s/ in isolation. The first strategy is to have the patient produce /θ/ and gradually reposition the tongue behind the front teeth to approximate /s/ placement. The patient can be verbally instructed in the following manner: "Let's make the /θ/. Keep making it and slide your tongue just behind your teeth. Listen for the difference in the sound when your tongue goes behind your teeth." The second strategy is having the patient articulate /t/ and then release the sound to make an /s/. The patient can also be directed to repeat /t/ and transition to an /s/ production /t-t-t-t-t-sssss/. Golding-Kushner (2001) recommends using a coarticulatory technique by presenting a word with /t/ in the postvocalic position. The patient is instructed to articulate a target word such as "pet" and to prolong the /t/ at the end of the word. This treatment strategy often results in the target production of "pets." Trost-Cardamone (2013) also discusses the use of speech sounds such as /f/ and /h/ to shape correct production of /s/. The /z/ can be elicited by cueing the patient to produce a sustained /s/ and then "turning on the speech motor," so that /z/ is produced /sssssszzzzzz/. Acquisition of the alveolar fricatives is an important milestone for the patient with cleft palate.

Velars

The velar point of articulation is the next to be introduced. The speech sounds /ŋ, k, g/ can be very difficult for some patients to acquire. Some patients experience difficulty acquiring correct production of the velar plosives /k, g/ because their placement is the most posterior in the vocal tract. This posterior point of articulation can trigger pharyngeal or glottal stop substitutions (Golding-Kushner, 1995). Therefore, Golding-Kushner recommends that the nasal /ŋ/ ("ng") be taught first. Keep in mind that /ŋ/ only occurs in the inter- and postvocalic word positions; it does not occur in the prevocalic position. A coarticulatory technique for /ŋ/ is to have the patient articulate the sound in the intervocalic position using the vowel /i/ as in "meet" as a juxtaposed sound (/iŋi/). Golding-Kushner (2001) reasoned that this context paired with the target sound minimizes the probability of triggering a more posterior articulation, since the vowel articulation involves a high front tongue position. When correct articulation of the target sound /ŋ/ is attained, the nasal can be used to achieve production of the voiced velar plosive /g/. To teach production of /g/, the patient can be instructed to "Make the sound with the back part of your tongue. Make it a long sound while I hold your nose." The SLP then uses an imitative model in the sequence /iŋgi-iŋgi-iŋgi/ for the patient to repeat. The patient is instructed to repeat the model with the nostrils occluded. Correct production is followed by a shift to the coarticulatory stimulus /iŋgi-gi/ with the nostrils occluded. After correct placement of /g/ is realized, practice transitions to syllable or word stimuli without occluding the nostrils. The /k/ is then presented and the patient is given a verbal placement cue such as "Make the /g/ sound but don't turn on your voice motor. Just let the air come out when you make the sound." In this section of teaching, the voiced plosive sound is taught initially rather than the voiceless-voiced sequence that has been followed. The rationale for this switch is a clinical hypothesis that patients with cleft palate have less trouble acquiring /g/ than /k/ and that the /ŋ/ is a coarticulatory facilitating agent for /g/.

Palatals

The last set of sounds in the teaching sequence are the palatal fricatives /ʃ, ʒ/ and the affricates /tʃ, dʒ/. These speech sounds are also pressure sounds and often misarticulated by patients with cleft lip and palate. Some teaching techniques for eliciting /ʃ/ include the following, instructing the patient as follows:

"I want you to pull your tongue back a little bit when you make /s/ so that you make /ʃ/." The movement of the tongue from /s/ to /ʃ/ is often a facilitating agent for patients (Riski, 2003; Trost-Cardamone, 2013). If necessary, the patient's nostrils can be occluded to enable sufficient oral air pressure impoundment. Kummer (2014) recommends that the patient be taught to produce a big sigh with the teeth closed but not clenched and lips rounded. The patient assumes the articulatory position, while being cued to "I want you to move your tongue until you make the whisper sound /ʃ/." Phonation prompts such as "I want you to turn on your motor and make the sound /ʒ/" can be employed following correct placement of /ʃ/. Similar to /ʃ/, it may be necessary to occlude the nostrils when attempting to produce /ʒ/ correctly. Note that integrating /ʒ/ into words will be in the inter- and postvocalic word positions.

Affricate speech sounds include production features of both stops and fricatives. There is a complete occlusion of the vocal tract followed by a sustained release. One teaching technique for /tʃ/ is to have the patient repeat /t-t-t-t-t/ and then shift the tongue tip to the palatal point of articulation for /tʃ/. Another sound elicitation technique is to instruct the patient to sneeze by starting with the mouth closed and then producing the /tʃ/ (Kummer, 2014). The voiced cognate /dʒ/ can be shaped in the same way as discussed with /ʒ/, if necessary.

Summary

A phonetic teaching sound-by-sound approach was described for the treatment of compensatory and maladaptive errors (Ruscello, 2017). It was recommended that different types of feedback information be utilized to create an awareness of the production features of the error versus the target sound. In some cases, verbal imagery was proposed to create an internal contrast between the compensatory error and the target sound. Order of sound treatment began with /h/ and then shifted to target sounds from an anterior to posterior point of articulation. Finally, different facilitating techniques were discussed to assist the patient with cleft palate in sound acquisition. Since a structural deficit is the causal agent in many treatment scenarios, the major aim is to change the place of articulation.

■ Additional Treatment Concerns

Liquids and Glides

The liquid and glide speech sounds /w, j, l, r/ were not discussed in the previous section. The rationale is that the sounds are voiced and do not require the generation of oral pressure. Nevertheless, these sounds may be produced with hypernasal resonance. Trost-Cardamone (1990a) wrote that the /l, r/ speech sounds are sometimes produced at a velar point of articulation by some patients with cleft palate. The /l/ → /ʟ/ and the /r/ → /ʀ/. The SLP should look and listen carefully for the possibility that the sounds may be articulated with a more posterior point of articulation. They also need to keep in mind that backing of liquids is seen in the speech of patients without velopharyngeal closure deficits. If identified, the errors should be subject to treatment but pressure-generating techniques like occluding the nostrils would not be necessary.

Lateralization

Lateralization is a nondevelopmental speech sound distortion that is articulated by directing the air stream off the sides of the tongue rather than using a central air stream. This type of error is present in the speech of patients without VPD; however, it has been noted clinically that many patients with cleft palate frequently produce lingual fricatives and affricates in a lateralized manner. Patients who have cleft palate and posterior crossbites or lateral open bites may lateralize lingual fricatives and/or affricates (Trost-Cardamone, 1990b; Zajac & Vallino, 2017). It is possible that lateralization in the presence of a malocclusion may be an obligatory error due to a presenting dental condition. However, dental or orthodontic correction of the malocclusion generally does not result in spontaneous elimination of lateralization. Consequently, treatment is needed to correct the problem. Riski (2003) recommends the release of /t/ to /s/ as described previously. Some SLPs use a coarticulatory facilitation technique to elicit a target sound. For instance, the patient is instructed to repeat the phrase "get you" quickly and then told to blend gradually the two words together so that the perceptual result is /tʃ/.

Cultural Considerations

The assessment and treatment of communication disorders in patients with clefts has been discussed; however, it should be noted that cultural considerations should also be taken into account for many patients (Moore, 2016). The population of the United States is composed of a diverse group of people with different cultural beliefs and values (Torres, 2013). With cleft palate, we are dealing with communication disorders secondary to a birth defect that involves facial disfigurement. Even if we feel that a family is acculturated, Torrres (2013) points out that families frequently withdraw to things that provide comfort and familiarity in times of emotionally charged situations. Understanding differences and how they play into the dynamics of family interactions is very important for the SLP to be cognizant of when providing services. Toliver-Weddington (1990) writes that the success of a treatment program for African American patients with cleft palate is a function of the family's sensitivity to the nature of the presenting cleft condition, the reasons or causes of the problem, and the prescribed treatment. Interactions with the family by the SLP should consider these factors when discussing and implementing the communication treatment plan. It is important that the SLP be aware of, respect, and integrate cultural sensitivity into the patient's care plan (Cheng, 1990; Myerson, 1990).

The attainment and maintenance of cultural competence is an ongoing process for the SLP who provides services to patients from diverse cultural backgrounds (ASHA, n.d.-a). The culturally competent SLP respects cultural differences and individual variations among patients, and examines her or his attitudes and beliefs toward different cultural groups. It also fosters the SLP's use of evidence-based practices within a context of cultural understanding. Moore (2016) presents an excellent discussion of evaluation and treatment considerations when working with Spanish-speaking patients presenting with cleft palate. The author discusses a number of tactics for assessment and treatment of patients speaking Spanish only and those with some English proficiency. The information is very informative and illustrates effective strategies for working with this population. SLPs are encouraged to access this work, if they provide services to culturally diverse patients of Latino origin.

Another population of patients who also require cultural understanding and competence on the part of the SLP are those who have undergone international adoption and present with cleft palate. Morgan, O'Gara, Albert, and Kapp-Simon (2016) examined the literature and reported a dearth of studies dealing with patients who present with cleft palate and have been internationally adopted. The authors indicated that services for these patients are often delayed, which places then at risk for speech and language problems. Based on their clinical experience, they suggest close monitoring of the patients in relation to their cognitive, motor, social, and communication development. Furthermore, it is recommended that the parents be educated in home stimulation techniques and the team SLP engage in collaboration with the patient's SLP and educational personnel in an effort to minimize the impact of any potential speech and/or language deficits.

Some major cultural considerations among African American, Latino, and Asian American groups have been identified in the literature and are summarized in Table 4–3. In addition, the web reference for the ASHA Position Statement on Cultural Competence in Service Delivery (2017) is included for reference.

■ A Technology for Treatment

In the current discussion, speech sound errors were characterized as primarily phonetic-based errors, and various treatment methods and procedures were discussed from that perspective. There are different theoretical positions that guide treatment for individuals with sound system disorders (Bernthal & Bankson, 2017). For example, we can use a motor skill learning (phonetic) perspective, or we might employ another treatment approach such as a cognitive-linguistic (phonemic)

Table 4–3. Major Cultural Variables Found Among African American, Latino, and Asian American Groups

Ethnicity	Cultural Awareness Variables
African American families	The SLP needs to be familiar with the dialect and culture of African Americans, which includes interacting with multiple family members and understanding that sometimes the cause of a cleft is attributed to folk beliefs. Often, family members feel that the SLPs are expert and rely on them to treat the child. Family is more disposed to participate when they feel that they can be of assistance. Interactional verbal and nonverbal behaviors to be aware of include: It is inappropriate to touch the hair or head of an African American. Speakers prefer indirect eye contact. Posing personal questions is considered to be improper. Avoid the use of direct questions. Interrupting a person during a conversation is acceptable.
Latinos	Make an attempt to understand the culture and beliefs of the family in regard to the cause and treatment of the child. If the SLP is not bilingual, an interpreter is necessary. Share information with the interpreter and provide in-service training if needed. The SLP needs to maintain eye contact with the patient/family during interactions with an interpreter. It is best not to use a family member for interpreting information. It is helpful to acquire some basic words/phrases in Spanish. Recommendations should be compiled into short simple lists for the family. The child's extended family can be a good resource for home treatment.
Asian Americans	SLPs need to recognize the cultural diversity among Asian/Pacific cultural groups. SLPs need to be aware of and respect the belief system of the child's family. Professionals are respected, so credibility is essential. The idea of seeking family input for a treatment plan may be perceived as a negative factor.

continues

Table 4–3. *continued*

Ethnicity	Cultural Awareness Variables
Asian Americans *continued*	Interactional verbal and nonverbal behaviors to be aware of include: Use open-ended questions rather than direct questioning. Avoid direct eye contact with family members. Discuss issues in a clear and concise manner. Make sure that the family members understand the information that is presented.

Note. Refer to ASHA Practice Portal—Cultural Competence in Service Delivery (http://www.asha.org/Practice-Portal/Professional-Issues/Cultural-Competence/).

approach. In comparing the two models, they are more alike than different, but the fundamental difference pertains to the teaching of rules. In motor learning, the SLP teaches practice units with the idea of generalizing a rule pertaining to the physical movements of the sound. That is, the purpose is to modify an existing motor pattern (substitutions, distortions). As previously discussed in this chapter, there is an implicit assumption that the target is part of the patient's phonological system, but it is not being used on the surface (Ruscello, 2008a). In motor learning, practice is used to form a motor skill that the SLP wants to incorporate into the patient's sound system. This is consistent with our position and that of other researchers (Golding-Kushner, 2001; Peterson-Falzone et al., 2017; Trost-Cardamone, 2013; Trost-Cardamone & Bernthal, 1993). Table 4–4 lists the components of the recommended teaching strategy that incorporates SLP-generated evidence of treatment (Byiers, Reichle, & Symons, 2012).

Treatment goals are developed from the results of assessment, which include the speech sound testing and spontaneous sample of conversation. Compensatory and maladaptive errors are identified and possible error patterns identified to determine what is to be taught. This is followed by the collection of a baseline, which tells the SLP if the selected targets are appropriate goals for therapy. A single-subject AB design can be used for the purpose of collecting a pretreat-

Table 4–4. Components of the Motor Learning Teaching Strategy

Component	*Process*
Content for treatment.	Select targets for treatment based on assessment.
Establish a pretreatment level of response.	Baseline target sounds prior to initiating treatment.
Develop a treatment paradigm.	Implement treatment using the principles of motor learning.
Monitor the child's response to the treatment.	Set response criterion and collect daily performance data. Assess for generalization.

ment baseline and probing the patient's speech behavior during the treatment period to validate a treatment effect (Byiers et al., 2012). The SLP needs to sample the behavior of interest in sufficient depth. Sampling tasks need to contain word items with the target sound(s) and items with target sound(s) in context. No reinforcement or performance information is given to the patient, since the target sound(s) is not yet being taught. The ideal baseline shows a stabile pattern of incorrect productions, which indicates that the patient is not producing the targets. The same pretesting items and procedures will be used for probes that are administered periodically during the course of therapy. It is expected that probe scores improve with treatment.

There are a number of implications that are associated with the motor learning approach to treatment. Generally, researchers indicate that a learner passes through different stages of motor skill development (Ruscello, 1993). Initially, it is conceptualized that the learner attempts to acquire a motor skill through activities that incorporate practice under conscious control. That is, the learner needs to "think" about what she or he is practicing. The learner is placed in a problem-solving situation that requires mental focus during practice. The motor skill is carried out in a restricted, self-guided mode with feedback and knowledge of results provided. Feedback is knowledge that the learner internalizes from her or his practice trials through various forms of sensory feedback and conscious introspection, while knowledge of results (KR) is that information of performance that is provided by an external source such as the SLP. The KR can be quantitative ("Good job!"), qualitative ("That's not right. Your tongue was sticking out!"), or both.

After the learner has carried out the skill through practice and conscious introspection, other practice activities are introduced to automate the skilled pattern (Ruscello, 2008a). The learner no longer needs to focus on the mental substrates of the skill but rather carries out the skill under a variety of conditions and practice contexts. The skill is becoming part of the learner's motor skill repertoire. Practice is a key ingredient in the process, and research suggests that distributed practice results in slightly better learning and retention than massed practice. This means that 3- to 30-minute sessions spread across 1 week would be more effective than one weekly session of 90 minutes.

Different types of practice are utilized and are presumed to be on a linguistic continuum of complexity. Remediation generally consists of a stair-step strategy, which progresses from isolation to conversational practice. Isolation, nonce or nonsense words, words, phrases, sentences, and conversational speech are used. Moreover, responses are elicited via imitation or evoked through more spontaneous procedures such as pictures or questions. In addition, there are several different ways to present practice items, and they may consist of either block or random sequencing. Block sequencing is most typical with material introduced that is similar. For instance, a patient is exposed to five to seven practice words that contain the target sound. The patient achieves correct target production for that material and is then exposed to the next practice condition. Random sequencing is different in that the patient is exposed to the practice items but the items may consist of five practice items with the target and five practice items without the target. The 10 items are presented in random order, and the patient is required to produce the targets presented randomly and the other items that do not contain the target sound. Table 4–5 presents some examples of presenting target items.

Table 4–5. Examples of Target Sound Presentation Via a Motor Learning Paradigm

Stimulus Presentation	Child's Response	Internal Feedback and Knowledge of Results
Example 1 "I want you to think about your new sound in the word. Remember to put your tongue behind your teeth for the /s/. Think about where you are putting your tongue and then say the word."	/sop/	"Good job!" (KR)[a] (Quantitative KR)
Example 2 "Say each picture after I say it." "Say the word _____."	/sop/	"Good job!" (KR) (Quantitative KR) "You made the 'tippie' sound and not the 'throaty' sound." (Qualitative KR)
Example 3 "I will show you a picture and I want you to say it."	/sop/	"Good job!" (KR) "You made your tongue work and not your voice box!" (Qualitative KR)
Example 4 "Tell me everything about this picture. What are the boys doing?"	/ðe brok ðə ' sas pæn/	"Great job!" (KR) (Quantitative KR) "You used your tongue when you said your new sound!" (Qualitative KR)
Example 5 "This is a /sri/ Say /sri/." The illustrated shape represents a nonce item. It is a nonword that is not phonologically permissible and used to reduce interference from the error sound, since it is unfamiliar to the child.	/sri/	"Good job!" (KR)

[a]KR stands for knowledge of results.

199

The SLP is advised to emphasize practice and to vary the stimuli to establish a strong motor pattern. For instance, the SLP may employ a variety of elicitation cues such as imitative cues ("Say ball"), delayed imitation ("This is a ball. What did I say?"), and spontaneous cues ("What is this?"). The SLP needs to provide clear and unambiguous information to the learner, so that she or he may benefit from feedback and KR. Similar to other therapy approaches, the SLP must monitor training trials and collect response accuracy data. Performance data for daily sessions should be at a level of 75% or higher (Ruscello, 2008a). Generally, we set a higher accuracy criterion in speech-language pathology that may range from 80% to 90%. If the patient's response accuracy levels drop below 75%, the data suggest that the treatment may be too difficult for the patient. Modifications in the teaching plan need to be made.

It is important to remember that the achievement of treatment goals is determined through the setting of completion criteria. When setting a criterion, the SLP can base it on either time or count. For instance, an SLP can set a response accuracy criterion at 90% accuracy for two blocks of 20 training trials. That is, the patient would need to produce correctly 18 of 20 stimulus presentations across two consecutive blocks of 20 training trials. Conversely, an SLP could have established a 90% rate of accuracy across a 15-minute segment of practice on a particular task. When the criterion is completed for the treatment task, the treatment step is completed and the patient moves to the next step. Daily performance percentages are maintained to ensure that the patient is responding to the treatment in a positive way. An example of data collection might look something like the following:

Daily Response Data	Date	Percentage of Accuracy
	2/4	81%
	2/6	78%
	2/9	91%
	2/12	88%
	2/14	89%

Finally, validating a treatment effect is a key factor of any viable treatment approach. It is important that the SLP generate patient performance data to show that the treatment has a positive influence on speech sound behavior. Validation of the data can be established through the collection of training trial data and response generalization. The training trial data consist of response accuracy data that have been collected for each treatment session in response to training trials. The other type of performance data is the patient's generalization or response to treatment outside of the treatment paradigm. Some SLPs refer to it as carryover. Following pretreatment baseline measures, probes are taken during therapy at 1- to 2-week intervals to determine if some change has taken place. This is the primary measurement component of the AB design that was discussed previously. A positive change in probe measures indicates that the patient is generalizing to untaught items and suggests that the treatment is an effective agent of change.

■ Summary

SLPs are educated and trained clinically to provide assessment and treatment services to patients with different speech and language disorders. Patients with VPD constitute a low-incidence group, and as a result, many SLPs do not work with this population on a frequent basis. A diagnostic plan for the perceptual assessment of patients with VPD was presented for use by SLPs, who do not have extensive experience in this clinical area. The components of the assessment are based on best practice recommendations that are contained in the literature (Henningsson et al., 2008). In some cases, the SLP will collect the pertinent data and work in collaboration with the patient's craniofacial team, while in other instances, the SLP will be collecting data for referral to a team. Treating the communication disorders of the patient will generally be the main focus of the local SLP. The treatment may be based on recommendations from the patient's craniofacial team SLP, or the plan may be developed and implemented by the patient's local SLP. In either event, the treatment strategies and teaching technology discussed herein provide the bases for modifying compensatory and maladaptive errors. The evidence base for such treatments is limited, but data do indicate treatment has resulted in positive change for patients with cleft palate who do and do not present with VPD (Bessell et al., 2013). In addition, the SLP needs to adapt assessment/treatment strategies in cases where cultural differences exist (Torres, 2013) and be cognizant of cultural differences that may need to be considered in the development and implementation of a treatment plan. Finally, concepts of motor learning were presented and recommended as the teaching technology or framework for delivering the phonetic treatment components that were discussed. For additional current information regarding different aspects of cleft care, the reader may also refer to http://www .asha.org/Practice-Portal/Clinical-Topics/Cleft-Lip-and-Palate/ (ASHA, n.d.-b).

5

Referring to a Cleft Palate–Craniofacial Team

Key Terms

- American Cleft Palate–Craniofacial Association (ACPA)
- Collaboration
- Collaborative Models
  - ☐ Parallel Delivery
  - ☐ Informal Consultation
  - ☐ Formal Consultation
  - ☐ Coprovision of Care
  - ☐ Collaborative Expansion
- Consent
- Health Insurance Portability Accountability Act (HIPAA)
- Interdisciplinary Team
- Referral Models
  - ☐ Active
  - ☐ Cold
  - ☐ Facilitated
  - ☐ Passive
  - ☐ Warm

■ Introduction

In this *Resource*, we listened to a variety of resonance and speech disorders associated with cleft lip and palate (CLP) and other problems of velopharyngeal dysfunction (VPD). The standard of practice for managing these disorders is interdisciplinary team-based care American Cleft Palate-Craniofacial Association (ACPA) Parameters for Evaluation and Treatment of Patients with Cleft Lip/Palate or Other Craniofacial Differences, 2018. Although most children with CLP receive the services of a team, there are some who do not or may have a speech problem for which VPD is suspect. The SLP who refers to a cleft palate team understands that the needs of his or her patient are very important. For many SLPs, however, making the referral to the team can be challenging. SLPs may be at a loss as to how and where to find a cleft palate team. A connected referral network, one that makes the referral process collaborative and barrier free, is key to ensuring best care for the patient. The focus of this chapter is to describe the elements of making a referral to a cleft palate team and a process for referral.

■ Overview of a Cleft Palate Team

CLP is a complex disorder that can manifest with a variety of different problems (i.e., speech, hearing, dental). Early on, the professionals treating those with CLP recognized that individually they were unable to provide for all the medical and psychosocial needs of these patients. They recognized that the best care for them is team care in which fragmented health care is converted to integrated health care (Nester, 2016). A team-based approach to care promotes communication and collaboration among the professionals caring for these patients to achieve quality care and positive outcomes. An interdisciplinary cleft palate team consists of specialists from different disciplines who work together to provide coordinated and comprehensive services to a patient with CLP and his or her caregivers. The specialists making up a team are listed in Table 5–1.

Why Refer to a Cleft Palate Team?

Referrals are made for a number of reasons: (1) to establish a diagnosis (i.e., VPD, posterior nasal fricative), (2) to determine treatment (e.g., speech therapy, surgery), (3) for further specialized testing using techniques that are unavailable to the clinician in the community (e.g., nasoendoscopy, pressure-flow testing), (4) for advice on management, and (5) for reassurance (Foot, Naylor, & Imison, 2010). Referral to a cleft palate team is a key part of the SLP's role in ensuring optimal care for the child or young adult with CLP.

Here are examples of some situations in which an SLP might refer a patient to a cleft palate team:

- The child with CLP who is being treated by an SLP in school or in a community-based program (i.e., Early Intervention) but who has not been routinely or consistently cared for by a team. A referral back to a team may be necessary to facilitate further treatment planning.
- The child who does not have overt signs of a palatal anomaly but who exhibits a speech disorder suggestive of possible VPD. In this instance, the SLP "hears" nasal speech or perceives the child's speech as atypical and significantly impaired enough to interfere with communication and questions the adequacy of velopharyngeal function.
- The SLP who believes that the patient's speech problem goes beyond his or her own experience or expertise. In this case, it is appropriate to seek consultation to rule out or confirm the clinician's assessment suspicions.

Table 5–1. The Cleft Palate-Craniofacial Team

Team Member	Role on the Team
Team coordinator	This person typically oversees the coordination of team care, reviews team recommendations, and ensures follow-up. The coordinator is most often the first point of contact between the referring SLP and the family or patient.
Orthodontist	Provides orthodontic treatment to reposition the teeth to optimize jaw relationships and occlusion and aligns malpositioned incisors and expands the maxillary arch to create an appropriate relationship with the lower dental arch. Fabricates presurgical infant orthopedics to reposition maxillary segments prior to lip repair.
Speech-language pathologist (SLP)	Provides family support and assistance for feeding the newborn with cleft palate. The SLP provides information concerning normal speech and language development, evaluates language and articulation skills. The SLP determines the nature of a speech disorder, if present, and the causative factors. The specialist may perform a variety of diagnostic tests to assess VPD. The SLP makes recommendations for treatment, monitors the effect of treatment, and routinely assesses communication progress.
Plastic surgeon	Plans and performs surgery including cleft lip repair, cleft palate repair, oronasal fistulae, pharyngoplasty (i.e., pharyngeal flap) to correct VPD, and nasal and lip revisions.
Otolaryngologist (ear, nose, throat [ENT] specialist)	Performs medical and surgical treatment of disorders of the ears, nose, and throat. The otolaryngologist manages ear infections, middle ear effusion (OME), and other problems of the outer, middle, and inner ear. He or she also manages upper airway problems and surgically remove the adenoids and tonsils.
Audiologist	Provides comprehensive hearing assessments, identifies hearing loss, and makes recommendations for treatment and follow-up services.
Geneticist and genetic counselor	The *geneticist* is a medical doctor who evaluates an individual and/or the family to diagnose, confirm, or rule out a genetic condition. The geneticist may recommend genetic testing that can help understand the cause and natural history of the disorder, and provides ongoing follow-up as needed.

Table 5–1. *continued*

Team Member	Role on the Team
Geneticist and genetic counselor *continued*	The *genetic counselor* is a health care professional (nonphysician) with specialized training in medical genetics and counseling who assesses a person or family about their risk for a variety of inherited conditions, genetic disorders, and birth defects and counsels them about the condition and how the diagnosis might affect other family members.
Pediatrician	A doctor who focuses on the physical, mental, and emotional health and well-being of a child at every stage of development. The pediatrician provides preventive health maintenance and medical care (short-term and long-term) for children.
Dentist	Provides continuous and comprehensive general dental care and promotes the maintenance of oral hygiene.
Oral maxillofacial surgeon	Plans and performs alveolar bone grafts to treat residual alveolar clefts and orthognathic (jaw) surgery to provide optimal relationships between the upper and lower jaws and adequate dental occlusion.
Prosthodontist	A dental specialist who focuses on the restoration of teeth and replaces missing teeth to improve appearance. The prosthodontist makes palatal devices for feeding and also fabricates prosthetic appliances such as a palatal lift or bulb to assist with velopharyngeal closure for speech.
Psychologist	The psychologist performs evaluations of development, learning, or adjustment when indicated. This specialist addresses behavior disorders or problems with emotional adjustment due to social difficulties that may arise secondary to a speech difficulty or facial difference.
Social worker	This professional helps individuals and their families to enhance their capacity for social functioning and assists them in overcoming various challenges in life. The social worker provides information related to cost of care and medical assistance and helps with identification of local agency assistance.
Patient and caregiver	The patient and caregiver are vital team members. They work together with team specialists to reach a decision about treatment and plan of care (shared decision making). Patients and caregivers play a key role in the medical decisions that affect their health.

When making a referral it is important for the SLP to avoid telling the family or patient that specific surgical or other treatment will be necessary to treat the speech problem, when in fact the suggested treatment is not indicated. For by doing so, it can cause disappointment and frustration for the caregivers and the patients themselves. Rather, best care for the patient is for the SLP to tell the family that the speech problem he or she hears is unfamiliar and would like to seek the opinion of a team of professionals to guide diagnosis and management.

■ The Referral Process

The referral process is an "active process of linking a person with a need or problem with a service which will meet the need or solve the problem" (Croneberger & Luck, 1985). Rather than being a matter of diverting care to someone else, referral is a systematic approach to obtain appropriate services to improve a person's current problem (Edwards, Davies, Ploeg, Virani, & Skelly, 2007). It involves transfer of trust from one clinician (i.e., community-based SLP) to another (i.e., cleft palate team SLP) to provide needed care that will better serve the patient because the problem (i.e., hypernasal speech) is beyond the level of the treating SLP's expertise.

It may be that some community-based SLPs perceive a gap between themselves and the team—a notion that can lead to barriers to care. The cornerstone to an effective referral process is collaboration (Young, 2000). Collaboration provides a holistic approach in effectively meeting patients' needs and helping them to move one step closer to addressing and resolving the problem. Grames (2004) suggested that most often the challenges experienced by these clinicians occur as a result of different perceptions of their roles and responsibilities regarding patient needs and the different goals they have for patient care. If the focus is kept on patient-centeredness and improving the person's quality of life, then the re-ferring SLP does not stop working with the patient but rather works as part of the team to optimally meet the patient's needs.

In cases where the SLP is unsure about a referral, a telephone consultation with the team SLP may help sort out relevant issues, explore alternate approaches or identify other resources to better serve the patient, facilitate a referral to the cleft palate team. By doing so, it ensures that the patient receives the necessary service and care. Perhaps the best that can be said is, when in doubt, refer.

There are several types of referral models available to the SLP that can facilate the patient's access to a cleft palate team. The approach to accessing a team can fall into one of five referral categories: passive, facilitated, active, cold, and warm ("Linking to other services," n.d.) (Table 5–2). Although each model has advantages and disadvantages, the common goal of any referral is to link the patient with the team, ensure a smooth process, and prevent the patient from falling through the cracks during the transition from the community-based SLP to the cleft palate team.

◼ Guidelines for Referring to a Cleft Palate Team

The often-asked questions by community-based SLPs are "How do I make a referral?" and "Where do I start?" The activities involved in a referral entail several processes to ensure best care for the patient. Figure 5–1 shows how these processes interact before, during, and after the referral to a cleft palate team is made.

The basic elements of a referral include ascertainment of consent to share information, locating a cleft palate team, accessing a cleft palate team, and communication between the referring SLP and the team. The SLP always needs to be mindful that the patient and/or patient's caregivers are involved in decision making around the referral (Foot et al., 2010). In other words, discuss openly and honestly about the referral and the reason for it.

Table 5–2. Types of Referral to a Cleft Palate Team

Type of Referral[a]	Characteristics	Advantages and Disadvantages
Passive referral	The patient[b] is given the contact information for the cleft palate team and is left to contact the team on his or her own time.	*Advantage*: Process gives the responsibility to patient to act on his or her own to contact the team for an appointment. *Disadvantage*: There is a greater likelihood that the patient will not make the call and follow up with the referral to the team.
Facilitated referral	The school-based SLP makes the arrangements with the cleft palate team on the patient's behalf and asks the cleft palate team coordinator to contact the patient.	*Advantage*: The SLP contacts the cleft palate team coordinator directly on the caregiver's behalf. *Disadvantage*: The patient has to wait for the team coordinator to contact him or her, and this could provide uncertainty as to when this contact may occur.
Active referral	The SLP contacts the cleft palate team coordinator or a member of the team with information about the patient. The coordinator typically contacts the patient for an appointment.	*Advantage*: The patient does not have to repeat the information about the problem or services already provided. *Disadvantage*: There is a risk that the information provided may have been miscommunicated or taken out of context.
Cold referral	The patient is referred to a service other than the cleft palate team.	*Advantage*: Perhaps no real advantage unless the referral is made for a condition for which there is no need for the services of a cleft palate team. *Disadvantage*: The person may be deprived of the appropriate team services for managing a speech disorder associated with VPD.

Table 5–2. *continued*

Type of Referral[a]	Characteristics	Advantages and Disadvantages
Warm referral	A three-way conversation via phone conference or videoconference that involves the community-based SLP, the team coordinator or SLP, and the caregiver/patient in which the referring SLP introduces the patient to the team coordinator or SLP and explains the case and reason for referral.	*Advantage:* The referral is an open and transparent process. Clarification of information can be made if needed. *Disadvantage:* Requires that all parties are available and have the means to participate in the communication. Among the five types of referral, this is perhaps the most infrequently used by the SLP.

Source: Modified with permission from: Linking to other services: referral guidelines for family relationship centres and the family relationship advice line. (n.d.). Retrieved February 7, 2017, from https://www.ag.gov.au/FamiliesAndMarriage/Families/Family RelationshipServices/Documents/Referral%20Guidelines.pdf

[a]Important note: The clinician is responsible for obtaining consent from the patient before making any team referral.

[b]In this table, we use the term *patient* to refer to caregiver of the child who is in need of service or the young adult who is managing his or her own care. We recognize that community-based SLPs or those working in academic settings refer to the patient as "client."

Consent

The Health Insurance Portability and Accountability Act (HIPAA, 1996) was established to protect the privacy of health information. To safeguard the patient's privacy, it is expected that consent be obtained before a referral to a cleft palate team is made. Consent is an integral aspect of service provision. It is an important process in which the person giving the consent is fully informed as to reason for the referral and of the information that will be provided to the team. For a child, the parents or legal guardians must sign a release authorizing the SLP to provide information to the team. In the United

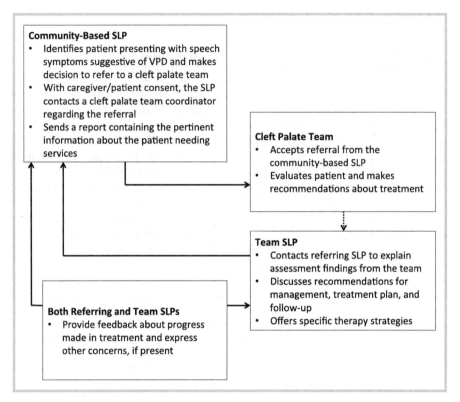

Figure 5–1. The referral process.

States, depending upon the state, the age of consent is between 16 and 18 years. These individuals can provide their own consent.

Locating a Team

In any case, when the SLP is going to refer, is unsure whether to refer, or would like to consider a referral and wishes first to speak to someone experienced in disorders of VPD, contacting a cleft palate team is encouraged. To locate a treatment team in a specific region, SLPs can visit the Cleft and Craniofacial Team Listings (http://acpa-cpf.org/team-care/team-listings/) on the ACPA website (http://acpa-cpf.org) or call the ACPA National Office at 1-800-24-CLEFT (25338). SLPs can then contact the local team and ask to speak with the clinical coordinator or SLP who serves on the team.

Communicating With the Team

When referring to a cleft palate team, the SLP making the referral should send a report with as much pertinent information as possible about the individual needing the service. This ensures that all parties are communicating and the process is well coordinated. There are three key points in making a referral to a cleft palate team: (1) Tell the team what you want from them, (2) do not be afraid to say you are unsure as to what the problem is, and (3) be clear and concise.

Briefly, the report should follow the general organization and format:

- *Patient identification (name, gender, date of birth).* Include diagnosis, if it is known (i.e., cleft lip and palate, developmental delay).
- *Reason for team referral and a description of concerns.* For example, the patient has a cleft lip and palate that has not been managed by a team. Or, the patient has a history of team management but has not had a team visit for the past 1 or more years. Or, your have concerns about hypernasal speech when the patient does not have an obvious cleft palate.
- *Statement about speech and symptoms.* Provide information about speech testing and results.
- *Relevant medical and developmental history.* If known, include information about hearing status, history of middle ear fluid treated with ventilation tubes and adenoidectomy, if known. If present, provide information about developmental differences.
- *Describe current speech therapy program.* Include what has been done so far such as frequency of services, goals, and progress. Attach a copy of recent test results, IEP plan, and written progress report. If the child has not been enrolled in speech therapy, state this as well.

A sample of a letter of referral to a cleft palate team is shown in Figure 5–2.

Somewhere Elementary School
123 4th Street
Somewhere, USA

10 April 2017

Somewhere Hospital Cleft Palate Team
Attn: Team Coordinator
456 Fixit Lane
Somewhere, USA

SUBJECT: Referral to Cleft Palate Team

Dear Ms. Smith,

Please accept this referral on Fiona Oppih, aged 5;1 years (DOB: 3/1/2012), for evaluation of resonance and velopharyngeal function due to concerns about hypernasal speech.

I recently saw Fiona during a speech screening at school. My findings revealed mild hypernasality and audible nasal emission. Mother indicated that she also hears a nasal tone in her daughter's speech. Fiona's articulation is within normal limits for age. Fiona currently attends kindergarten and is performing well in class. There are no developmental concerns. To date, Fiona has not received speech therapy.

Fiona does not have an overt cleft palate. However, upon oral examination I noticed a bifid uvula. She has a history of middle ear fluid treated with ear tubes. Mother reported that she noticed Fiona seemed to hear better following tube placement. Fiona underwent an adenoidectomy approximately one year ago with no reported change in her speech. Family history is negative for speech and hearing problems.

I have discussed my findings and recommendations with the mother who indicated that she is interested in a referral to your team in order to learn more about Fiona's speech problem. I have given her your phone number and she will be contacting you for an appointment.

Please call me at 123-456-7890 if you have questions. I look forward to hearing about your assessment findings and recommendations and working with you to help Fiona improve her speech.

Thank you for your attention to this referral.

Sincerely,

Eleanor Nella, MS, CCC-SLP

Figure 5–2. Sample referral letter to a cleft palate team.

■ After the Referral Is Made: What Can the SLP Expect From the Team?

After the referral to a cleft palate team has been made and the patient has been evaluated by the specialists on the cleft palate team, the referring SLP should expect to be contacted by the team SLP to discuss the visit outcome. This follow-up communication should take place within 1 to 3 weeks after the team visit and may be in the form of a direct phone call or a written report. During this communication, the team SLP will explain the assessment findings in detail, discussing those factors contributing to the speech problems (i.e., occlusal defects, hearing loss, suspected velopharyngeal dysfunction). The team SLP will clearly discuss recommendations for management (i.e., speech therapy, imaging of the velopharyngeal mechanism, ventilation tubes), and a plan for follow-up (Daly & Wilson, 2015). It should be expected that the strategies recommended for remediating articulation errors (if needed) are evidence based. The team SLP should also offer to provide appropriate literature and handouts to facilitate treatment.

Grames (2004) aptly states that good communication and collaboration among the local and team SLPs (and other team members) "is the best tool that we have for power sharing and quality care provision" (p. 7). There are available collaborative techniques that can be effective based on the needs of the child and constraints of the situation. Lorenz and colleagues (2009) describe five collaboration models: parallel delivery, informal consultation, formal consultation, coprovision of care, and collaborative networking. Table 5–3 presents these collaborative models described by Grames (2004) for use in the care of patients with CLP.

The specific collaborative model used will depend on the needs of the patient, the caregivers, the purpose of collaboration, and the recommendations of the SLPs. The benefit of this open communication during collaboration is that it enhances care, bridges the perceived gap between the team and local SLPs, and most of all provides the best care possible for the patient.

Table 5–3. Collaborative Models That May Be Used to Facilitate Communication Between the Referring and Team Speech-Language Pathologists

Models of Collaboration	Key Components
Parallel delivery	Each SLP is responsible for a certain aspect of the patient's treatment. There is no overlap in service provision.
Informal consultation	A consultant SLP provides guidance to the school SLP concerning the child's communication disorder. The SLP may never have face-to-face contact with or even know the patient.
Formal consultation	The team SLP provides diagnostic services, which are communicated to the school SLP for implementation. It is a cooperative venture between the two entities.
Co-provision of care	The team SLP and school SLP share common treatment goals. They meet periodically to discuss progress and implement various agreed upon modifications in the treatment plan.
Collaborative expansion	There is an expansion of the collaborative team to include other medical and educational specialists who may assist in achieving certain care goals. The child's parents may also be enlisted to help with the care plan.

Source: Reprinted with permission from Ruscello, D. M. (2017). School-based intervention. In D. Zajac & L. Vallino (Eds.), *Evaluation and management of cleft lip and palate.* San Diego, CA: Plural Publishing.

■ Summary

An SLP who suspects a speech problem suggestive of VPD should refer his or her patient to a cleft palate team. For some SLPs, making the referral to a team can be a bit of a mystery. This chapter provided information about the referral process and underscored the importance of collaboration between the community-based SLP and the cleft palate team. The components of a referral letter to the cleft palate team were outlined and an example of a letter presented. We also discussed what the community-based SLP can expect from the team SLP after the team visit and the importance of collaborative care.

APPENDIX A

Audio Case Studies:
Analysis of Speech and
Treatment Recommendations

Audio Case Study 3.3.1

This is a 20-year-old male with repaired bilateral cleft lip and palate.

Case History

Surgical: Tracheostomy in the newborn period for subglottic stenosis and was cannulated at 1 year of age. Lip repair at 9 months, palate repair at 19 months, and a superiorly based pharyngeal flap to correct VPD at age 5 years. Myringotomy and pressure equalization (PE) tubes to manage otitis media with effusion (OME) in the past.

Dental: Severe skeletal Class III malocclusion with open bite. This patient is currently preparing for maxillary advancement (LeFort I osteotomy) using distraction osteogenesis (MADO).

Hearing: An audiological evaluation completed at the time of this assessment showed normal hearing sensitivity, bilaterally.

Speech Therapy: History of speech therapy in elementary school. During this visit, this young adult expressed no concerns about his speech.

 Listen to Audio 3.3.1.

Speech Assessment:

Resonance: WNL

Nasal air emission: None apparent (NA)

Articulation: Fronting of the palatal fricatives and affricates

Phonation: WNL

Impression of Speech: Speech is suggestive of adequate velopharyngeal function. The patient presents with essentially normal speech. There is fronting of the alveolar and palatal sounds, but they are minor obligatory distortions due to the Class III occlusal relationship, which do not adversely affect speech intelligibility.

Recommendations: It is necessary to follow this patient and monitor speech skills particularly following maxillary advancement. Successful advancement would create an oral environment conducive to tongue-alveolar and tongue-palatal contact; however, in some cases, patients develop velopharyngeal dysfunction (VPD) following significant advancement of the maxilla. (Clinical note: Since this recording, the patient underwent maxillary advancement using distraction osteogenesis. Resonance was unchanged and remained normal afterward.)

Audio Case Study 3.3.2

This is a 12-year-old male with repaired left cleft lip and palate and history of left maxillary collapse. Mirror testing showed no visible nasal air emission. He has no history of speech therapy.

 Listen to Audio 3.3.2.

Speech Assessment:

Resonance: Slightly hyponasal

Nasal air emission: NA

Articulation: Lateralization of the alveolar and palatal fricatives and affricates

Phonation: WNL

Impression of Speech: This patient is slightly hyponasal and lateralizes a number of sounds. He is intelligible but the identified errors are nondevelopmental distortion errors (/s, z, ʃ, ʒ, tʃ, dʒ/) that are evident in the patient's speech, most likely associated with his occlusal defect.

Recommendations: Monitor the patient through the cleft palate team and enroll in a trial of treatment to correct the lateral emission errors. Keep in mind that the presence of the left maxillary collapse may preclude complete amelioration of the speech errors through speech therapy alone. Speech may improve after correction of the maxillary structural defect, and if it does not improve, speech therapy would then be warranted.

Audio Case Study 3.3.3

This is a 7-year-old male with repaired bilateral cleft lip and palate.

Case History

<u>Surgical</u>: The lip was repaired at 3 months, the palate at 14 months, and a sphincter pharyngoplasty at age 6 years.

<u>Dental</u>: He presents with a narrow premaxillary segment that will require correction.

> **Listen to Audio 3.3.3.** *Note.* In this audio, you will hear the SLP providing speech prompts.

Speech Assessment:

   Resonance: Mild to moderate hypernasality

   Nasal air emission: NA

   Articulation: Lateralization of the alveolar and palatal fricatives and affricates (/s/, /z/, /ʃ/, and /tʃ/)

   Phonation: WNL

<u>Impression of Speech</u>: Both resonance and speech sound production errors are present in the patient's speech sample.

<u>Recommendations</u>: Monitor the patient for any future needs through the cleft palate team, which would include instrumental assessment of velopharyngeal function and treatment of the premaxillary arch restriction. Trial speech treatment to correct the lateral distortions of /s, z, ʃ, ʒ, tʃ, dʒ/ may be a consideration. The presence of the oral structural defect may preclude complete amelioration of the speech errors through speech therapy alone. Speech may improve after correction of the maxillary structural defect, and if it does not improve, speech therapy would then be warranted.

Audio Case Study 3.3.4

This is a 9-year-old male with Stickler syndrome and repaired cleft palate. His features include mandibular hypoplasia and myopia (near sightedness) for which he wears glasses and hearing loss. Throughout the years, the caretaker had considered this child's speech to be acceptable even though hypernasality had been documented during previous routine team visits. More recently, she expressed concerns about the child's nasality.

Case History

Surgical: At 2 months of age, he underwent mandibular distraction osteogenesis to improve the airway and cleft palate repair at 10 months.

Dental: Class II malocclusion

Hearing: An audiological evaluation completed at the time of this assessment showed a mild to moderate sensorineural hearing loss (SNHL) in the right ear and a mild to moderate mixed hearing loss 250 to 6000 Hz sloping to profound at 8000 Hz in the left ear. The family is not interested in pursuing amplification.

Speech Therapy: Attended private speech therapy as a toddler but was no longer enrolled at the time of this visit.

 Listen to Audio 3.3.4.

Speech Assessment:

Resonance: Mild to moderate hypernasality

Nasal air emission: Nasal emission that is most distinctive on voiceless plosives

Articulation: There is a slight /s/ distortion and inconsistent /r/ distortion.

Phonation: WNL

<u>Impression of Speech</u>: Speech is intelligible but hypernasality is present. Minor errors of /s/ and /r/ are present in the speech sample as is intermittent audible nasal emission. The nasal emission is present most often during production of plosive sounds.

<u>Recommendations</u>: It is important that the patient continue to be seen by the cleft palate team for the purpose of developing a management plan that meets the patient's needs and is acceptable in this case to the caregiver. The child presents with speech, resonance, and dento-skeletal issues that require comprehensive management. Instrumental assessment of velopharyngeal function using imaging studies and pressure-flow testing may be considered if the patient and his family are interested in correcting VPD. Hearing should also be monitored routinely. Although the caregiver is presently not interested in pursuing amplification, preferential seating toward the front of the classroom at school is supported.

Audio Case Study 3.3.5

This is an 11-year-old female with 22q11.2 deletion syndrome who was referred to the cleft palate team due to concerns regarding hypernasality. She does not have a cleft palate.

Case History

Surgical: None to date

Dental: Class I incisal relationship

Hearing: An audiological evaluation completed at the time of this assessment showed normal hearing, bilaterally.

Speech Therapy: She has a history of speech and language therapy, and experiences some learning challenges. Based on the IEP, the current focus of speech therapy is on the remediation of /k, g/ and /s/.

 Listen to Audio 3.3.5.

Speech Assessment:

    Resonance: Mild hypernasality

    Nasal air emission: NA

    Articulation: Speech sound errors with /s, r, θ/

    Phonation: Mild hoarseness

Impression of Speech: The patient presents with resonance, articulation, and phonatory problems, which appear to be mild in severity. The sample shows inconsistent error production of /r/ and more consistent errors with /s/, including cluster reduction and occasional final consonant deletion, and /θ/ is also misarticulated.

Recommendations: A complete phonetic/phonemic analysis is recommended to identify the residual error patterns displayed by the child, so that a revised treatment plan can be implemented. This can be done by the patient's school SLP and shared with the team SLP. Periodic perceptual and instrumental management by the team SLP should be conducted along with any other needs of the patient. Would not consider management of the VPD at this time.

Audio Case Study 3.3.6

This is an 11-year-old male with a repaired left unilateral cleft lip and palate. This was his first visit with the cleft palate team.

Case History

Surgical: The cleft lip and palate were repaired but a left maxillary cleft remains and requires repair.

Dental: Mixed dentition and dental crowding. Class III relationship with anterior and bilateral posterior crossbite. The palate appears short in the anterior-posterior dimension.

Hearing: History of otitis media with effusion treated with myringotomies and PE tubes. Mild low-frequency conductive hearing loss in the left ear and normal hearing in the right ear.

Speech Therapy: Currently enrolled in speech therapy for correction of /s/ and /z/.

 Listen to Audio 3.3.6.

Speech Assessment:

    Resonance: Mild hypernasality

    Nasal air emission: Intermittent audible nasal air emission

    Articulation: Within functional limits

    Phonation: Within normal limits

Impression of Speech: The patient presents with mild hypernasality and satisfactory oral sound placement for all speech sounds with the exception of the /s, z/ speech sounds. Productions of the alveolar fricatives were perceived as oral distortions of the intended targets. Intermittent mild audible nasal emission was noted during the production of /s/ target items. From the audio alone, it is difficult to tell if the nasal air escape is obligatory or learned.

<u>Recommendations</u>: Monitor the patient for any future needs through the cleft palate team, which would include instrumental assessment of velopharyngeal function, since secondary management of velopharyngeal function might be a future consideration for this patient.

Audio Case Study 3.3.7

This 4-year-old female was referred by her otolaryngologist for an assessment of velopharyngeal function for speech.

Case History

<u>Surgical</u>: No surgical history

<u>Hearing</u>: An audiological evaluation completed at the time of this assessment showed normal hearing, bilaterally.

<u>Speech Therapy</u>: The child has a history of speech therapy to correct articulation errors.

 Listen to Audio 3.3.7.

<u>Speech Assessment:</u>

Resonance: WNL

Nasal air emission: There is some mild nasal turbulence during the production of /dʒ/ and /tʃ/ (in "Jimmy" and "Charlie") as part of the posterior nasal fricatives.

Articulation: Posterior nasal fricatives (PSNE) on affricates

Phonation: WNL

<u>Impression of Speech</u>: Most plosives are produced normally and there is no hypernasal voice quality. The child produced posterior nasal fricatives characterized by nasal turbulence for affricates. Although produced without salient nasal turbulence, the child's production of oral stops as replacements for /s/ and /z/ is likely part of a pattern of posterior nasal fricatives.

<u>Recommendations</u>: SLPs who do not see children with cleft palate on a frequent basis should be alert to PSNE. When present, be sure to assess all pressure sounds, because the child

with VPD will experience problems with all pressure sounds and resonance will be hypernasal. In this case, the nasal fricatives were limited to sibilants and affricates. This is a case of mislearning and it requires treatment by an SLP. Referral to a cleft palate team is not necessary.

Audio Case Study 3.3.8

This is a 15-year-old male with popliteal pterygium syndrome, cleft palate, lip pits on the lower lip, and left choanal atresia with recurrent nasal congestion. There is a fistula at the junction of the hard and soft palate approximately 2 mm wide and 3 to 4 mm in length. He has a history of OME treated with PE tubes.

Case History

Surgical: Palate repair at 8 months. The choanal atresia was repaired, resulting in improved airflow through the nose.

Dental: Deep vertical overbite

Hearing: An audiological evaluation completed at the time of this assessment showed that hearing sensitivity is essentially within normal limits for the left ear, with a slight hearing loss noted at 250 and 6000 Hz, and a slight conductive hearing loss present from 1000 to 2000 Hz in the right ear.

Videonasoendoscopic Assessment: Videonasoendoscopy showed a coronal pattern of velopharyngeal movement with a large central gap. These findings were discussed with the caregiver and patient, who indicated that he is currently not interested in treatment to correct his VPD.

 Listen to Audio 3.3.8.

Speech Assessment:

Resonance: Moderate hypernasality

Nasal air emission: Audible nasal air emission with /s/

Articulation: /s/ is produced with nasal emission, glottal stops are present in the postvocalic position, and the palatal fricatives and affricates are fronted.

Phonation: WNL

<u>Impression of Speech</u>: Speech is intelligible but the audible nasal emission and hypernasality are very prominent features of the patient's speech and do call attention from listeners.

<u>Recommendations</u>: Although he does not wish to pursue any management of VPD at this time, periodic appointments with the cleft palate team should be continued to include perceptual and instrumental measures of speech production and resonance. Would consider management of the VPD, if the patient wished to pursue that option.

Audio Case Study 3.3.9

This is a 17-year-old female with repaired right unilateral cleft lip and palate. She has a history of maxillary advancement, resulting in increased nasality.

Case History

<u>Surgical</u>: Maxillary advancement to correct malocclusion, after which she reported experiencing occasional nasal reflux.

<u>Oral Examination</u>: A well-formed Passavant's ridge was observed.

<u>Pressure-Flow Studies</u>: Findings showed estimated velopharyngeal areas that ranged from 12 to 38 mm^2 depending upon the speech sample.

 Listen to Audio 3.3.9.

<u>Speech Assessment</u>:

    Resonance: Mild hypernasality

    Nasal air emission: Intermittent audible nasal emission

    Articulation: WNL

    Phonation: WNL

<u>Impression of Speech</u>: Patient is intelligible with satisfactory oral placements but hypernasality and occasional nasal emission are present in the sample.

<u>Recommendations</u>: Periodic perceptual and instrumental assessments by the cleft palate team SLP should be conducted along with any other needs of the patient. Would consider management of the VPD, if the patient wished to pursue that option.

Audio Case Study 3.3.10

This is a 6-year-old female with repaired bilateral cleft lip and palate. She has maxillary alveolar clefts that will be repaired. She has a history of OME and hearing loss.

Case History

Surgical: Lip repair at 4 months and palate repair at 11 months

Dental: Class III bilateral posterior crossbite

Hearing: An audiological evaluation completed at the time of this assessment showed a mild conductive hearing loss at 250 and 500 Hz rising to normal hearing from 1000 to 8000 Hz, bilaterally.

Speech Therapy: History of speech therapy beginning with Early Intervention. She continues to receive this service through the school district.

> ### Listen to Audio 3.3.10.

Speech Assessment:

Resonance: Moderate hypernasality

Nasal air emission: Intermittent audible nasal emission

Articulation: Compensatory and obligatory errors

Phonation: WNL

Impression of Speech: This patient presents with hypernasality and compensatory (e.g., glottal stops) and obligatory (e.g., nasalized plosives) speech errors, which collectively interfere with speech intelligibility.

Recommendations: Behavioral treatment is recommended and should be directed to the variability in the child's consonant inventory. In particular, glottal stops that appear to be used inconsistently for oral consonants should be targeted. Nasal emission is an obligatory symptom and would not be targeted in behavioral therapy. Periodic perceptual and instrumental assessments by the team SLP should be conducted along with any other needs of the patient. Physical management of the VPD is an important component of the patient's treatment plan and should be a primary goal of the team.

Audio Case Study 3.3.11

(*Note.* This case is also presented in Video 3.4.6.)

This is an 18-year-old female with repaired left unilateral cleft lip and palate. She first presented to the cleft palate team at age 7.

Case History

Surgical: Palate repaired at 12 months

Dental: She is in active orthodontics and has a Class I incisal relationship.

Hearing: She has a history of OME and hearing loss.

Pressure-Flow Studies: Findings showed estimated velopharyngeal orifice areas that exceeded 20 mm^2, consistent with inadequate velopharyngeal closure.

Imaging Studies: Multiview videofluoroscopy and videonasoendoscopy confirmed VPD.

Speech Therapy: No known history of speech therapy

> ### *Listen to Audio 3.3.11.*

Speech Assessment:

Resonance: Moderate hypernasality

Nasal air emission: Audible nasal emission

Articulation: Weak pressure consonants

Phonation: WNL

Impression of Speech: This patient's speech is suggestive of velopharyngeal dysfunction on the basis of the perceptual findings of moderate hypernasality, weak pressure consonants, and audible nasal air emission and instrumental assessments.

<u>Recommendations</u>: Pharyngoplasty to correct velopharyngeal dysfunction to eliminate or reduce hypernasality was recommended. Of note, the patient chose to have the procedure. Based on the imaging studies, the surgeon elected to do push-back revision palatoplasty with buccal flaps.

Audio Case Study 3.3.12

This is an 8-year-old female with Stickler syndrome and repaired isolated cleft palate. She reported that her classmates have a difficult time understanding her. It is worth noting that for the past several years, this child had been scheduled for instrumental assessment of velopharyngeal function but the parents did not keep the appointments.

Case History

Surgical: Palate repaired at 11 months. PE tubes to manage OME were inserted at the time of palate repair. Tubes were replaced at age 5 years.

Dental: Mixed dentition with a left posterior crossbite and Class I occlusion

Hearing: An audiological evaluation completed at the time of this assessment showed normal hearing, bilaterally.

Pressure-Flow Studies: Findings showed estimated VP areas of 7.2 mm^2 on /p/ in "hamper" with complete overlap of oral pressure, nasal pressure, and nasal airflow during /mp/ segments. Recorded mean nasal airflow rate on /p/ in syllables was 149 mL/s. These results are consistent with incomplete velar closure.

Speech Therapy: She has never been enrolled in speech therapy.

Listen to Audio 3.3.12.

Speech Assessment:

Resonance: Mild hypernasality

Nasal air emission: Nasal turbulence is present on fricatives and stops.

Articulation: WNL

Phonation: WNL

<u>Impression of Speech</u>: The patient exhibits satisfactory oral placements but moderate hypernasality and nasal turbulence are present. Turbulence is particularly evident in alveolar /s/ and /t/ word contexts. It is fairly consistent but not on every high-pressure segment. Intelligibility is within functional limits (WFL).

<u>Recommendations</u>: Follow-up with instrumental studies of velopharyngeal function and development of a plan to manage the VPD.

Audio Case Study 3.3.13

This is a 13-year-old male with Klippel-Feil syndrome and repaired left unilateral cleft lip and palate who was first seen by the team at age 7 years. He also has microcephaly, hearing loss for which he wears hearing aids, and learning challenges. He also wears glasses. He has limited nasal airflow through both nostrils.

Case History

Surgical: Lip and palate surgery was done elsewhere. The timing of surgery is unknown.

Dental: Class III incisal relationship and mixed dentition. He wears a maxillary holding appliance.

Hearing: An audiological evaluation completed at the time of this assessment showed a moderately severe rising to essentially slight conductive hearing loss in the right ear and a moderate rising to essentially mild conductive hearing loss in the left ear. He wears binaural hearing aids.

Speech Therapy: He has a history of speech and language therapy beginning with early intervention. He continues to receive this service at school. The mother reported that the focus of treatment is on rate reduction.

> ***Listen to Audio 3.3.13.***

Speech Assessment:

Resonance: Hyponasal

Nasal air emission: NA

Articulation: Fronting of alveolar sounds and /r/ distortion. He has an /ng/-like substitution for /n/.

Phonation: WNL

Impression of Speech: The patient is hyponasal and note in the above description the documented nasal airflow problem. He is fronting the alveolar and palatal sounds due to the Class III occlusion. He has a residual /r/ problem and a very unusual substitution of the nasal /n/. During productions of /n/, particularly in the counting task, a /g/ is perceived, but in some cases, it is perceived as an /n/ immediately followed by /g/. When he produced the word "wagon," the /n/ was substituted by /g/.

Recommendations: Recommend treatment of the residual /r/ and /g/ substitution. The effect of the hearing loss on these errors cannot be overlooked, and therefore this patient should continue to wear his hearing aids in therapy to assist in the treatment. The fronting errors are obligatory and need to be monitored as he undergoes treatment for the malocclusion. Periodic perceptual and instrumental assessments by the team SLP should be conducted along with any other needs of the patient, including study of the hyponasality.

Audio Case Study 3.3.14

(*Note.* This child is also presented in Video 3.4.12.)

This is an almost 8-year-old male with repaired bilateral cleft lip and palate who was internationally adopted at 15 months of age. He has a history of OME and hearing loss.

Case History

Surgical: Cleft lip was repaired in the country of birth prior to adoption. Palate repair at 17 months after he joined his family. Myringotomy and PE tubes inserted at the time of palate repair.

Dental: Early mixed dentition. Skeletal Class III. There is an anterior crossbite and a left crossbite in the canine and first molar region.

Hearing: An audiological evaluation completed at the time of this assessment showed a mild low-frequency conductive hearing loss, bilaterally.

Speech Therapy: Started speech therapy through Early Intervention and is currently receiving treatment at school and hospital-based programs to correct articulation errors.

Pressure-Flow Studies: Findings showed estimated VP areas exceeding that of 20 mm² on /p/ in "hamper" with complete overlap of oral pressure, nasal pressure, and nasal airflow during /mp/ segments.

> ### Listen to Audio 3.3.14.

Speech Assessment:

Resonance: Moderate hypernasality

Nasal air emission: When the child is not using major compensations such as the /s/ in "Sissy sees the sky," there is some ANE.

Articulation: Lateralization of /s, z, ʃ, ʒ, tʃ, dʒ /, variable glottal stop for /k/

Phonation: WNL

Impression of Speech: Speech intelligibility is limited in this patient due to the hypernasality and speech production errors. The patient is producing the alveolar and palatal fricatives and affricates with lateral emission. Glottal stop substitution is variable for /k/ in the post- and intervocalic position of words.

Recommendations: Recommend continuing speech therapy to correct the errors that were present in the speech sample. Follow-up with imaging studies of velopharyngeal function and development of a plan to manage the VPD.

Audio Case Study 3.3.15

(*Note*. This child is also presented in Video 3.4.9.)

This is an almost 7-year-old female with neurofibromatosis 1 (NF1) who was referred by her school-based SLP to the cleft palate–craniofacial team because of concerns about hypernasal speech. She does not have a cleft palate.

Case History

(Additional information about this child's medical background is provided in the history for Video 3.4.9.)

<u>Surgical</u>: Tonsillectomy and adenoidectomy to relieve obstructive sleep apnea symptoms, but this was not helpful and she continues to experience the condition.

<u>Dental</u>: Missing central and lateral incisors

<u>Hearing</u>: An audiological evaluation completed at the time of this assessment showed normal hearing, bilaterally.

<u>Speech Therapy</u>: She was enrolled in Early Intervention until age 3 years, after which she attended a school for children with special needs in an integrated and developmentally appropriate setting until age 5 years. She is in Grade 1, where she receives physical, occupational, and speech therapies.

<u>Studies of Velopharyngeal Function</u>: Pressure-flow studies showed estimated mean areas on /p/ in syllables and "hamper" that exceeded 20 mm². Imaging of the velopharyngeal port using multiview videofluoroscopy and videonasoendoscopy showed very little palatal movement and lateral pharyngeal wall movement during phonation, resulting in a large velopharyngeal gap (see videonasoendoscopic assessment in Video 3.4.9).

Listen to Audio 3.3.15.

Speech Assessment:

Resonance: Severe hypernasality

Nasal air emission: Audible nasal air emisson

Articulation: Imprecise articulation

Phonation: Pitch variation

Impression of Speech: This child exhibits motor speech characteristics, demonstrating severe hypernasality, imprecise articulation, and abnormal pitch variations.

Recommendations: There are several factors of this child's medical condition that need to be considered in making the choice between surgery or a palatal lift (prosthesis) to improve resonance. There are several contraindications to surgery, including her complex medical condition, particularly her obstructive sleep apnea and the little to no movement of the velum and lateral pharyngeal walls observed during the imaging procedures. A palatal lift is recommended. Continued speech therapy is also recommended, which focuses on strategies to improve speech intelligibility. If intelligibility does not improve following the fitting of a lift and trial therapy, an augmentative assessment is recommended.

Audio Case Study 3.3.16

This is an almost 4-year-old male with repaired left unilateral cleft lip and palate who was internationally adopted at 21 months of age, after lip repair only. The palate was unrepaired. He has a history of OME and conductive hearing loss.

Case History

Surgical: Cleft lip was repaired in the country of birth prior to adoption. Palate repair at 22 months after he joined his adoptive family.

Dental: Anterior crossbite

Hearing: An audiological evaluation completed at the time of this assessment showed normal hearing, bilaterally.

Speech Therapy: Started speech therapy through Early Intervention and is currently receiving treatment at school to correct articulation errors.

Listen to Audio 3.3.16.

Speech Assessment:

Resonance: Moderate hypernasality

Nasal air emission: Audible nasal air emission

Articulation: Consistent use of glottal stops for plosives, pharyngeal stop on /k/, and developmental distortion on /r/ distortion.

Phonation: Severe hoarseness

Impression of Speech: Intelligibility is severely limited due to resonance, articulation, and phonatory disorders. The articulation errors include nasal fricatives and glottal stops, and in some cases, there are sound deletions. Hard glottal attack is present in a number of the utterances, particularly in the environment of stops. Hoarse voice quality is significant.

<u>Recommendations</u>: Recommend continuing speech therapy to treat the sound errors that were identified in the speech sample; however, a complete phonetic/phonemic analysis should be undertaken to identify all sound pattern errors. Follow up with instrumental studies of velopharyngeal function and formulate a plan to manage the VPD. The patient should also be seen for a laryngeal examination and treatment initiated per direction of the team otolaryngologist.

Audio Case Study 3.3.17

(*Note.* This child is also presented in Video 3.4.11.)

This 6-year-old female was referred to the cleft palate team by her school-based speech-language pathologist because of hypernasal speech and the presence of a bifid uvula. During her team visit, the surgeon confirmed a diagnosis of submucous cleft palate based on the findings of a bony notch in the posterior hard palate and partial zone of lucency in the midline.

Case History

Surgical: None to date

Dental: Class I occlusion

Hearing: No history of OME. An audiological evaluation completed at the time of this assessment showed normal hearing, bilaterally.

Speech Therapy: At the time of this visit, she has not received speech therapy.

> ### *Listen to Audio 3.3.17.*

Speech Assessment:

Resonance: Moderate hypernasality

Nasal air emission:

Articulation: Nasal fricative, /r/ error

Phonation: Mild hoarseness

Impression of Speech: The patient presents with hypernasality, speech sound errors, and mild hoarseness. Intelligibility is mildly impaired due to the multiple factors that are present in the patient's speech.

<u>Recommendations</u>: Recommend continuing speech therapy to correct the /s/ nasal fricative error that was present in the speech sample. The /r/ speech sound would not be a target due to developmental concerns. Follow up with instrumental studies of velopharyngeal function and formulate a plan to manage the VPD. Monitor vocal quality.

Audio Case Study 3.3.18

(*Note.* This child is also presented in Video 3.4.16.)

This is a 3.5-year-old male with repaired right unilateral cleft lip and palate who was internationally adopted at 32 months.

Case History

Surgical: The lip was repaired in the country of birth (date unknown) and the palate was repaired at 33 months, 1 month after his adoption. Myringotomies and PE tubes inserted at the time of palate repair.

Dental: Class I molar relationship

Hearing: An audiological evaluation completed at the time of this assessment showed a mild conductive hearing loss in the left ear and normal hearing in the right ear.

Speech Therapy: The patient was enrolled in speech therapy after the palate was repaired and continued to receive this service at the time of this assessment. The focus of treatment was to achieve correct articulatory placement for oral consonants and eliminate compensatory articulation errors associated with cleft palate.

Listen to Audio 3.3.18.

Speech Assessment:

Resonance: Moderate hypernasality

Nasal air emission: Audible nasal air emission

Articulation: Compensatory speech errors and a developmental speech error

Phonation: WNL

<u>Impression of Speech</u>: Intelligibility is limited due to the hypernasality, audible nasal emission, and compensatory speech errors, particularly glottal stops. Nasal emission is associated more frequently with the fricative sounds, while the glottal stops are used more in plosive contexts. There is also an /r/ error present but, at the patient's age, it is a developmental variation that would not be a speech target and it is not a pressure sound.

<u>Recommendations</u>: A home program should be initiated with this patient to develop consistent oral articulations, while developing the consonant inventory and increasing vocabulary. Plosives can be targeted initially and then fricatives and affricates. Since this patient is an adoptee from another country, higher-level language concepts should also be introduced. Treatment can also include simple closure techniques such as holding the nose to allow for the generation of adequate oral pressure requisite to pressure sound production. Training for the parents is necessary as is coordination of services with the community-based SLP. Monitor the patient for any future needs through the cleft palate team, which would include instrumental assessment of velopharyngeal function, since in all likelihood, secondary management of velopharyngeal function will be needed.

Audio Case Study 3.3.19

(*Note.* This child's speech was recorded before surgery to correct VPD. You will hear his audio in 3.3.20, one year after surgery.)

This is a 9-year-old male with repaired right unilateral cleft lip and palate. He was internationally adopted at almost 3 years of age.

Case History

Surgical: The cleft lip and palate were repaired in the child's country of birth before his arrival to this country. He underwent maxillary alveolar cleft repair at age 8 years.

Dental: Mixed dentition and Class III malocclusion

Hearing: History is positive for OME treated by myringotomy and PE tubes and fluctuating conductive hearing loss when the OME was present. At the time of this assessment, hearing was within normal limits bilaterally.

Speech Therapy: He has a history of speech therapy and currently receives this service at school to remediate his presenting articulation errors.

> ### *Listen to Audio 3.3.19.*

Speech Assessment:

Resonance: Mild hypernasality

Nasal air emission: NA

Articulation: Compensatory errors, including pharyngeal fricatives and affricates and glottal stops

Phonation: WNL

<u>Impression of Speech</u>: This patient's error pattern consists primarily of compensatory errors. The alveolar and palatal fricatives and affricates are produced at the pharyngeal point of articulation, and a majority of stops are articulated as glottal stops.

<u>Recommendations</u>: Continue speech therapy to correct the compensatory errors that were present in the speech sample. Follow up with instrumental studies of velopharyngeal function and formulate a plan to manage the VPD.

Audio Case Study 3.3.20

(*Note.* This is an audio of the child presented in Audio 3.3.19 one year after surgery to correct VPD. He is now 11 years old.)

Case History

Surgical: At age 10 years, this patient underwent pushback revision palatoplasty with buccal flaps to correct VPD.

Dental: Class III malocclusion and anterior crossbite

Hearing: Within normal limits, bilaterally

Speech Therapy: History of speech therapy to correct articulation errors and continues to receive this service in school

> ### Listen to Audio 3.3.20.

Speech Assessment:

Resonance: WNL

Nasal air emission: NA

Articulation: Glottal stops are corrected after surgery but pharyngeal fricatives were still substituted for /s/. Pharyngeal productions are also perceived on /ʃ/, and /tʃ/ but are less salient than perceived on the /s/ segments.

Phonation: WNL

Impression of Speech: Resonance improved after surgery and is judged to be within normal limits. The pharyngeal fricatives noted before surgery persist after surgery.

Recommendations: Continue speech therapy to correct the compensatory errors that are present in the speech sample. A motor learning approach to treatment is recommended, including awareness and discrimination until he achieves carryover to natural contexts, particularly with glottal stop productions (see Ruscello & Vallino, 2014).

Video Case Studies:
Analysis of Speech and
Treatment Recommendations

Video Case Study 3.4.1

This is a 2-year-old female with repaired complete cleft of the secondary palate.

Case History

<u>Surgical</u>: Palate repair at 12 months. OME treated with myringotomy and PE tubes at the time of palate repair.

<u>Hearing</u>: Responses to stimuli presented in sound field were within normal limits for at least the better ear.

<u>Speech Therapy</u>: Not enrolled in speech therapy

 Watch Video 3.4.1.

<u>Speech Assessment</u>:

Resonance: WNL

Nasal air emission: None apparent (NA)

Nasal grimace: None

Articulation: WNL

Phonation: WNL

<u>Impression of Speech:</u> Resonance is within normal limits. This child is producing oral pressure consonants /p, b, t, d, k, g/. Developmental substitutions include d/g and k/g—errors unrelated to the cleft palate. Phonation is within normal limits for age and gender. Overall, speech is suggestive of adequate velopharyngeal closure for speech at this time.

<u>Recommendations</u>: There are no specific recommendations for speech and language intervention; it is currently not warranted. Home speech and language stimulation activities to facilitate speech and language development are supported. Routine monitoring of speech, language, and hearing per cleft palate team and/or at the parents' request will be carried out.

Video Case Study 3.4.2

This is a 6-year-old male with repaired isolated cleft of the secondary palate.

Case History

Surgical: Palate repair at age 10 months. OME treated with myringotomy and PE tubes.

Dental: Mixed dentition. Class II relationship on the right, Class I on the left.

Hearing: Minimal mild sensorineural hearing loss at 2000 Hz, bilaterally. Normal middle ear function in both ears.

Speech Therapy: History of speech therapy to improve articulation

Watch Video 3.4.2.

Speech Assessment:

Resonance: WNL but hyponasality was noted in the sample

Nasal air emission: NA

Nasal grimace: None

Articulation: Developmental errors

Phonation: WNL

Impression of Speech: Resonance is considered to be WNL, though slight hyponasality was perceived. Phonation is also judged to be WNL. Articulation is characterized by /r/ distortions, fw/θw (e.g., "three"). These errors are unrelated to the cleft palate and classified as developmental errors.

Recommendations: Speech therapy is recommended to remediate articulation errors, since the youngster is 6 years of age. Speech, language, and hearing will be routinely monitored as per cleft palate team and/or at the parents' request.

Video Case Study 3.4.3

This is a 14-year-old female with repaired left unilateral cleft lip and palate. She was internationally adopted at age 5 years, following lip and palate repair. She first presented to the cleft palate team at age 6. During the most recent team assessment, however, they reported that hypernasality has become more noticeable during conversational speech and that the teachers notice it as well. This teen indicated that she is aware of the nasality and is interested in improving her speech.

Case History

Surgical: Lip and palate repair done in her country of birth. A remaining fistula in the hard palate was repaired after she joined her family. Alveolar cleft repair at age 9 years.

Dental: Maxillary expansion was completed prior to alveolar cleft repair. Orthodontic treatment is complete. She currently presents with a Class I occlusal relationship.

Hearing: Within normal limits, bilaterally

Speech Therapy: She has an extensive history of speech therapy that focused on the remediation of compensatory articulation errors, including pharyngeal fricatives and affricates. These errors have been corrected. She continues to receive speech therapy twice monthly to monitor articulation. It is worth mentioning that she also presented with palatalized /t/ and /d/, but these were spontaneously eliminated after maxillary expansion.

Studies of Velopharyngeal Function: Videonasoendoscopy was used to image the velopharyngeal port when the speaker was 10 years old. At that time, findings showed asymmetrical palatal elevation with robust closure noted on the right side and incomplete closure on the left side. The gap was judged to be small, with bubbling emanating from the port. An adenoid pad was present.

Watch Video 3.4.3.

Speech Assessment:

Resonance: Within functional limits (WFL) during sentence citation. Resonance breaks down during conversational speech when she becomes mildly hypernasal.

Nasal air emission: Audible nasal air emission during conversation with turbulence perceived on "put and baby" in "Put the baby in the buggy"

Nasal grimace: Occasional and slight

Articulation: In general, articulatory placement is good, particularly during sentence production when she reduced her speaking rate. However, during conversation when she used her typical rate, some pressure consonants are not produced correctly due to a lack of oral pressure.

Phonation: WNL

Nasoendoscopic Assessment: Findings show a pattern of asymmetrical closure with velopharyngeal elevation and closure on the right side and a gap on the left side. Note bulkier appearance of the muscle on the right side that contributed to closure on that side. There was some limited degree of lateral pharyngeal wall movement. When she produces phrases and sentences, you can observe bubbling at the open portion of the velopharyngeal port. You can observe a Passavant's pad as the patient moves toward closure but the bulging appears below the level of velopharyngeal closure. A final interesting feature is that you see a very distinctive contrast in the degree of closure when observing the client's pattern of closure during phrase and sentence repetition versus spontaneous conversational speech. The degree of port closure is greater for word and phrase repetition than spontaneous conversation.

Impression of Speech: This speaker's articulation and resonance were judged to be within functional limits (WFL) in citation, but resonance breaks down when she uses her typical rate during conversational speech, at which point nasal turbulence and weak oral pressure on oral pressure consonants can be perceived. The findings found on nasoendoscopy confirm VPD.

Recommendations: Based on perceptual and imaging studies, and considering the patient's desire to improve her speech, surgery to correct VPD is recommended.

Video Case Study 3.4.4

This is a 6-year-old male with repaired right unilateral cleft lip and palate.

Case History

<u>Medical</u>: Oral exam showed a short velum with good elevation during phonation and a Passavant's ridge.

<u>Surgical</u>: Lip repair at 3 months of age; palate repair at 9 months of age; secondary Furlow palatoplasty at approximately 5 years of age

<u>Dental</u>: Early mixed dentition, reverse overjet, and alveolar cleft

<u>Hearing</u>: Within normal limits, bilaterally

<u>Speech Therapy</u>: Currently enrolled in speech therapy

> ### *Watch Video 3.4.4.*

<u>Speech Assessment</u>:

Resonance: Mild hypernasality

Nasal air emission: Mild audible nasal air emission

Nasal grimace: Present

Articulation: Oral distortions on fricatives. Mandibular deviation to the right side during articulation, most noticeable on /s/ segments.

Phonation: WNL

<u>Impression of Speech</u>: The patient's speech is characterized by mild hypernasality, reduced loudness, audible nasal air emission, and weak pressure consonant production. In addition, articulation is marked by inconsistent oral distortions. Mild mandibular deviation to the right side was observed during speech production tasks. Overall speech is suggestive of inadequate velopharyngeal function.

<u>Recommendations</u>: Monitor the patient for future needs through the cleft palate team, which would include instrumental assessment of velopharyngeal function, because secondary management of velopharyngeal function will be necessary. Speech treatment may be directed to the mandibular deviation and stabilizing oral points of articulation through nostril occlusion. Occluding the nostrils will enable the patient to develop adequate oral pressure in treatment and in preparation of managing the VPD.

Video Case Study 3.4.5

This is an 11-year-old male with repaired bilateral cleft lip and palate. Attendance to the cleft clinic has been irregular.

Case History

<u>Surgical</u>: Lip repair was done at 3 months and palate closure at 12 months. An alveolar bone graft was done at 9 years of age.

<u>Dental</u>: Class III occlusion with a lateral crossbite

<u>Hearing</u>: At the time of testing, hearing was within normal limits, bilaterally.

<u>Speech Therapy</u>: The patient has received speech treatment but is no longer enrolled.

<u>Studies of Velopharyngeal Function</u>: Pressure-flow studies showed reduced oral pressure in the range of 3 to 5 mm^2 in the presence of concomitant nasal air pressure and airflow. Videonasoendoscopy showed a coronal pattern of velopharyngeal movement with a large central gap.

Watch Video 3.4.5.

<u>Speech Assessment</u>:

Resonance: Mild hypernasality

Nasal air emission: Audible nasal air emission

Nasal grimace: Present

Articulation: Obligatory oral distortions

Phonation: Hoarse vocal quality

<u>Impression of Speech</u>: Speech is characterized by mild hypernasality, audible (passive) nasal air emission, and nasal grimace, suggesting velopharyngeal dysfunction. Articulation is

marked by dentalized sibilants attributed to the Class III mal-occlusion and lateral crossbite. The patient also has a hoarse voice quality.

<u>Recommendations</u>: If there are no medical contraindications, a pharyngoplasty is recommended to improve velopharyngeal function and eliminate hypernasality and audible nasal air emission. The obligatory articulation errors are not amenable to speech therapy until the occlusal defect is corrected and in some cases spontaneously remediate as a function of an improved oral environment. Referral to the team otolaryngologist for a laryngeal voice examination and, if recommended, subsequent management of the voice problem is recommended.

Video Case Study 3.4.6

(*Note*. This is the same case presented in Audio 3.3.11. In this video, she is seen in before and after surgery to improve speech and resonance.)

This is an 18-year-old female with repaired left unilateral cleft lip and palate. She first presented to the cleft palate team at age 7, at which time resonance was judged to be within functional limits. Speech assessments over the course of subsequent team visits revealed gradual changes in resonance. Pressure-flow studies confirmed this change over time. However, the family and patient were reluctant to proceed with surgery to correct VPD until this recent assessment, when the patient reported that she was entering college and would like to sound better.

Case History

Surgical: Lip repair at 5 months and palate repair at 12 months. The maxillary alveolar cleft repair is completed. Pushback revision palatoplasty with buccal flaps at age 18 to correct VPD.

Dental: Currently in active orthodontics. Class I incisal relationship.

Hearing: Mild conductive hearing loss at 4000 to 6000 Hz in the right ear and a moderate to mild conductive hearing loss at the specific frequencies 250, 1000, and 4000 Hz in the left ear.

Speech Therapy: No known history of speech therapy

Studies of Velopharyngeal Function: Pressure-flow studies showed estimated mean areas on /p/ in syllables and "hamper" that exceeded 20 mm^2. Imaging of the velopharyngeal port using both multiview videofluoroscopy and videonasoendoscopy revealed incomplete velar closure and minimal lateral pharyngeal wall movement, resulting in a coronal pattern of velopharyngeal closure.

Watch Video 3.4.6.

Speech Assessment:

Parameters	Before Surgery	After Surgery
Resonance	Moderate hypernasality	Normal
Nasal air emission	Audible	Not perceived
Nasal grimace	Present	Not observed
Articulation	WNL	WNL
Phonation	WNL	WNL

Impression of Speech: Before surgery, this patient's speech is suggestive of VPD on the basis of the perceptual findings of moderate hypernasality, weak pressure consonants, and audible nasal air emission. Instrumental assessments confirmed VPD. After surgery, resonance is judged to be normal.

Recommendations: Surgery was successful in eliminating the speech symptoms associated with VPD. There are no specific recommendations for additional intervention. Continued follow-up for other cleft related issues is supported.

Video Case Study 3.4.7

This is an 11-year-old male who, at age 8, first presented to the cleft palate team due to concerns about hypernasal resonance. He does not have a cleft palate. The mother reported that her son, as a toddler, sounded nasal. Oral examination revealed asymmetrical velar movement during the production of /a/. Videonasoendoscopy confirmed palatal asymmetry. Findings showed robust velopharyngeal closure on the left side and incomplete closure on the right side. Surgery to correct VPD was done when he was 9 years old, after which the mother reported an improvement in resonance. Recently, however, this child requested a speech reevaluation because he perceived an increase in his nasality, and the mother agreed.

Case History

<u>Surgical</u>: Adenoidectomy at 2 years of age with no reported noticeable change in resonance. Two sets of PE tubes to treat OME. Pharyngoplasty with fat graft to the posterior pharyngeal wall at age 9.

<u>Dental</u>: Class III occlusion. He is currently wearing a quad helix, an orthodontic appliance used to widen the upper jaw.

<u>Hearing</u>: Within normal limits, bilaterally.

<u>Speech therapy</u>: History of speech therapy from kindergarten through third grade.

Watch Video 3.4.7.

<u>Speech Assessment</u>:

Resonance: During citation, resonance is mildly hypernasal but becomes moderately hypernasal during conversational speech.

Nasal air emission: Nasal turbulence noted occasionally during conversational speech.

Nasal grimace: None noted

Articulation: Oral distortions on sibilants associated with his malocclusion

Phonation: Mild-moderate hoarseness

<u>Impression of Speech</u>: Speech is suggestive of VPD.

<u>Recommendations</u>: Based on perceptual findings, and considering the patient's concern about his speech, nasoendoscopic reassessment of velopharyngeal is recommended in order to examine the integrity of the fat graft and to develop a treatment plan to manage this child's hypernasal speech.

Video Case Study 3.4.8

This is a 15-year-old male with Crouzon syndrome with maxillary hypoplasia. He is scheduled to undergo mandibular advancement and LeFort I osteotomy for maxillary advancement using distraction osteogenesis (MADO).

Case History

Medical: He has a history of obstructive sleep apnea, snoring, and mouth breathing.

Surgical: Cranial vault expansion with fronto-orbital advancement at age 3 years. Tonsillectomy and adenoidectomy at 13 years.

Dental: Skeletal Class III malocclusion. He has undergone orthodontic preparation for surgery. He currently is wearing braces.

Hearing: Within normal limits, bilaterally.

Watch Video 3.4.8.

Speech Assessment:

   Resonance: Mildly hyponasal

   Nasal air emission:

   Nasal grimace:

   Articulation: Fronting of sibilants and frictionalization on the double stops while counting 60 to 70 associated with the Class III malocclusion.

   Phonation: WNL

Impression of Speech: Audible breathing, hyponasal speech, and articulation errors are associated with this individual's midface hypoplasia and occlusal defect. Sound placement can be considered to be within functional limits.

<u>Recommendations</u>: There are no specific recommendations for speech at this time. Resonance and articulation will be reevaluated after surgery.

Video Case Study 3.4.9

(*Note.* This is the same case presented in Audio 3.3.15.)

This 6-year-old female with inherited NF1 was referred to the cleft palate–craniofacial team by her school-based SLP because of concerns about hypernasal speech. She does not have a cleft palate.

Case History

Medical: History is also significant for chemotherapy at 21 months for bilateral optic gliomas (she is blind in the right eye), seizure disease, and Moyamoya disease (a rare, progressive blood vessel or vascular disorder in which the carotid artery in the skull becomes blocked or narrowed, reducing blood flow to the brain). She has obstructive sleep apnea (OSA). She does not have a history of ear disease or hearing loss. She does not have any difficulty with nasal regurgitation.

Surgical: Right parietotemporal craniotomy to treat stenosis arteries associated with Moyamoya disease at 21 months. Tonsillectomy and adenoidectomy done to relieve OSA but it did not relieve the symptoms and OSA persists.

Dental: Missing central and lateral incisors

Hearing: At the time of testing, hearing was within normal limits, bilaterally.

Speech Therapy: Received Early Intervention until age 3 years and attended a school for children with special needs in an integrated and developmentally appropriate setting when she was 4 and 5 years old. She is currently a first grader and receives physical, occupational, and speech therapies.

Studies of Velopharyngeal Function: Pressure-flow studies showed estimated mean areas on /p/ in syllables and "hamper" that exceeded 20 mm^2. Imaging of the velopharyngeal port using both multiview videofluoroscopy showed very little palatal movement and lateral pharyngeal wall movement during phonation, resulting in a large velopharyngeal gap.

Watch Video 3.4.9. *Note.* In this conversational speech sample, the child is talking about the movie *Frozen*.

Speech Assessment:

Resonance: Severe hypernasality

Nasal air emission: Transient audible nasal emission on fricatives; may be difficult to perceive

Nasal grimace: Not observed

Articulation: Imprecise articulation

Phonation: Pitch variations

Nasoendoscopic Assessment: Findings showed limited velar movement during speech, resulting in a large central velopharyngeal gap. A significant feature of this examination is the right carotid artery pulsation.

Impression of Speech: The resonance feature and imprecise articulation are characteristics of dysarthria.

Recommendations: There are several factors of this child's medical condition that need to be considered in making the choice between surgery or a palatal lift (prosthesis) to improve resonance. There are several contraindications to surgery, including her complex medical condition, particularly her obstructive sleep apnea and the little to no movement of the velum and lateral pharyngeal walls observed on nasoendoscopy. A palatal lift is recommended. Continued speech therapy is also recommended, which focuses on strategies to improve speech intelligibility. If intelligibility does not improve following the fitting of a lift and trial therapy, an augmentative assessment is recommended.

Video Case Study 3.4.10

(*Note.* This is the same case presented in Audio 3.2.11.)

This is an 8-year-old female who was referred to the cleft palate team by the school-based speech-language pathologist because of concerns about nasal resonance. She has low muscle tone and some learning challenges.

Case History

<u>Medical</u>: The team surgeon diagnosed a submucous cleft palate on the basis of a bifid uvula, partial zone of lucency in the midline, and a small notch in the posterior hard palate. This child also has a history of OME.

<u>Surgical</u>: None to date

<u>Dental</u>: Open-bite malocclusion associated with a thumbsucking habit

<u>Hearing</u>: Recently received PE tubes to treat otitis media. Before tube insertion, she exhibited a mild bilateral conductive hearing loss. At the time of testing, hearing was within normal limits, bilaterally, after tubes.

<u>Speech Therapy</u>: Enrolled speech therapy

<u>Pressure Flow Studies</u>: Findings showed no differences in nasal and oral air pressures, suggestive of velopharyngeal inadequacy.

> ### *Watch Video 3.4.10.*

<u>Speech Assessment</u>:

Resonance: Mild to moderate hypernasality

Nasal air emission: Audible air emission

Nasal grimace: Not observed

Articulation: Developmental, residual, and maladaptive errors

Phonation: WNL

Impression of Speech: This is a very interesting patient who displays a number of different speech disorders. She presents with mild hypernasality during the recitation tasks, but the severity of the hypernasality increases during conversational speech. She fronts the alveolar and palatal sounds consistently with very visible tongue fronting caused by the open malocclusion. She also substitutes /f/ in place of /θ/. Pressure sounds produced with appropriate placement are produced with weak pressure. Note that during some productions of pressure sounds, nasal turbulence is audible. Also note that in some /s/ productions, she produces a nasal fricative rather than the lingual fronted production that she generally produces. In addition, there is a real difference between word production and conversational speech. When the patient engages in conversational speech, intelligibility is decreased.

Recommendations: Recommend speech therapy to correct the speech sound errors that are exhibited by the patient. Perceptual and instrumental studies of velopharyngeal function need to be carried out in order to develop a management plan to correct the VPD.

Video Case Study 3.4.11

(*Note.* This case was also presented in Audio 3.3.17.)

This is a 6-year-old female who was referred to the cleft palate team for issues related to resonance. The team surgeon confirmed the diagnosis of submucous cleft palate.

Case History

Surgical: None to date

Medical: Bifid uvula, partial zone of lucency in the midline, and a small notch in the posterior hard palate; findings consistent with submucous cleft palate. No history of OME.

Dental: Class I molar relationship

Hearing: At the time of testing, hearing was within normal limits, bilaterally.

Speech Therapy: At the time of this assessment, she had never been enrolled in speech therapy.

> ### *Watch Video 3.4.11.*

Speech Assessment:

   Resonance: Moderate hypernasality

   Nasal air emission: NA

   Nasal grimace: Present

   Articulation: Developmental and maladaptive errors

   Phonation: WNL

Nasoendoscopic Assessment: There is limited movement of the lateral pharyngeal walls and some movement of the velum toward approximating velopharyngeal closure for speech. A moderately sized central velopharyngeal gap with a coronal pattern is present throughout the speech sample. There is never a time in the sequence where the child moves toward complete closure. The most distinctive feature is the lack of levator muscle bulk at midline. Note the notch (or trough) on the nasal surface of the velum, a classic feature of a submucous cleft palate.

Impression of Speech: This patient presents with a number of articulation errors and hypernasal resonance. She produces a posterior nasal fricative for /s/. During /s/ productions, note that she also makes a dentalized tongue contact or complete tongue protrusion; however, it is difficult to discern if there is an oral and nasal coproduction as the major perceptual feature is the nasal production. The presence of posterior nasal fricatives was verified when her nose was held and she tried to prolong /s/. Note that she did produce an oral /s/ once when her nose was held, indicating that she is stimlable for the alveolar /s/. She also uses the stopping process for other oral sibilants on a variable basis, and fronting of those sounds is also seen inconsistently.

Recommendations: Speech therapy for the remediation of the posterior nasal fricatives and oral stopping and fronting processes. Barring any medical contraindications, this patient requires a surgical approach to manage the submucous cleft palate and VPD.

Video Case Study 3.4.12

(*Note.* This is the same case presented in Audio 3.3.14.)

This is an almost 8-year-old male with repaired bilateral cleft lip and palate who was internationally adopted at 15 months of age. History is significant for OME and associated hearing loss.

Case History

Surgical: Cleft lip was repaired in the country of birth prior to adoption. Palate repair at 17 months after he joined his adoptive family. Myringotomy and PE tubes inserted at the time of palate repair.

Dental: Early mixed dentition. Skeletal Class III. Anterior crossbite and a left crossbite in the canine and first molar region. Bilateral maxillary alveolar clefts with oronasal fistulas are present, but the child is not yet ready for maxillary expansion and bone graft to close to alveolar cleft.

Hearing: At the time of testing, he exhibited a mild low-frequency conductive hearing loss, bilaterally.

Speech Therapy: This child started speech therapy as part of an Early Intervention program and continued when he entered school. He is currently receiving treatment at school and also through a hospital-based program to correct articulation errors associated with the cleft.

Pressure-Flow Studies: Findings showed estimated VP areas exceeding that of 20 mm^2 on /p/ in "hamper" with complete overlap of oral pressure, nasal pressure, and nasal airflow during /mp/ segments.

Watch Video 3.4.12.

Speech Assessment:

Resonance: Moderate hypernasality

Nasal air emission: Audible nasal emission

Nasal grimace: Present

Articulation: Obligatory errors, compensatory errors

Phonation: WNL

Impression of Speech: Moderate hypernasality, audible nasal air emission, mild nasal grimace, and oral distortions (obligatory errors) characterized by palatalization of sibilants and stop consonants (i.e., /t/) associated with his midface hypoplasia. There were several interesting features of this child's speech. When counting from 60 to 70, he replaced /sk/ with /t/ and when producing 80 during counting from 80 to 90, he replaced /t/ with /d/. There is no correct placement for /f/. During more controlled contexts such as counting or sentence repetition, he produces perceptually accurate oral stops. However, during connected speech, he produces compensatory speech errors, particularly glottal stops. Note the production of /y/ for /z/ in "zoo." Phonation is unremarkable.

Recommendations: This patient requires a treatment plan that requires careful coordination among team members to treat the presenting speech and resonance problems. In terms of speech, a motor learning approach to treatment is recommended, including awareness and discrimination until he achieves carryover to natural contexts, particularly with glottal stop productions. However, the dental/occlusal problems present with this patient also present a challenge and must be managed by the orthodontist and oral surgeon. There needs to be an oral environment that supports correct lingual placement, thus minimizing the presence of obligatory placement errors. In addition, imaging the velopharyngeal valving mechanism during correct speech productions is needed to provide information needed to develop an optimal plan for managing velopharyngeal closure.

Video Case Study 3.4.13

This is an almost 7-year-old male with a repaired submucous cleft palate and history of OME. He first presented to the cleft palate team at 4 years old upon the referral of the otolaryngologist. This diagnosis of submucous cleft palate was based on the presence of a bifid uvula, translucent zone in the midline of the soft palate, and a notch in the posterior hard palate.

Case History

Surgical: Palate repair at 5 years. OME treated with myringotomy and PE tubes at the time of palate repair.

Dental: Class II occlusion

Hearing: At the time of testing, hearing was within normal limits, bilaterally.

Speech Therapy: Enrolled for the first time in speech therapy at age 4 years prior to team visit and continues to receive these services to correct articulation errors.

> ### *Watch Video 3.4.13.*

Speech Assessment:

    Resonance: Mild hypernasality

    Nasal air emission: NA

    Nasal grimace: Present, albeit slight

    Articulation: Primarily compensatory errors

    Phonation: NA

Impression of Speech: Although this child exhibits mild hypernasality, the most salient features about this child's speech are the productions of pharyngeal fricatives, especially for /s/ and glottal stops for /g/ and /t/. They are most prominent during connected speech and has a significant impact on intelligibility. He has good placement for bilabial plosives. Last, listen to the hard glottal attacks on vowels, particularly when they are adjacent to /b/.

<u>Recommendations</u>: Speech therapy that focuses on correcting the compensatory errors is recommended along with continued monitoring by the cleft palate team.

Video Case Study 3.4.14

This is a 3-year-old male with repaired left unilateral cleft lip and palate.

Case History

Surgical: Lip repair at 3 months and palate at 12 months. Myringotomies and PE tubes to treat OME done at the time of palate repair.

Dental: Class III and posterior crossbite. Missing left lateral incisor. Maxillary alveolar cleft repair will be done during the mixed stage of dentition between 7 and 10 years.

Hearing: At the time of testing, he exhibited a mild-moderate conductive hearing loss in speech frequency range in at least one ear and Type B tympanometric configurations bilaterally, suggestive of middle ear pathology. This child is scheduled to have his PE tubes replaced.

Speech Therapy: Enrolled in speech therapy

Watch Video 3.4.14.

Note. This child is producing words from the Arizona Articulation Proficiency Scale-2. A list of the words he is producing is provided to facilitate your understanding (few are completely unintelligible as shown by ??). He also produces a few spontaneous comments during the test.

Words: horse, nine, tree, cup, bath, comb, TV, cook, stove, ladder, ball, yellow, vanilla, bird, fork, ??, car, ear, ring, trees, ??, green, watch, zipper, nose, nest, carrot, books, cake, wagon

Speech Assessment:

    Resonance: Cannot judge at this time

    Nasal air emission: NA

Nasal grimace: Present

Articulation: Developmental and compensatory errors

Phonation: Hoarse vocal quality

<u>Impression of Speech</u>: This is an example of a child who has coexisting speech errors. Not all of his errors are related to velopharyngeal dysfunction. Speech sound production is characterized by numerous errors that include both compensatory and developmental errors. For example, articulation is marked by m/n substitution, h/k in "cup" and "comb." Note this child's tendency to want to occlude his nose during speech. This is what he learned to do in speech therapy. A pharyngeal fricative can be heard on the /s/ in "stove." Developmental w/l in "ladder." There is no bilabial placement for /b/ in "ball." For this case, it is important to undertake both a phonetic and phonemic analysis to establish the patient's phonetic and phonemic inventories. This would be of great assistance in the planning and implementation of a comprehensive treatment plan to improve speech sound production and overall language skills.

Note that this patient exhibits a nasal grimace. He also presents with moderate-severe hoarse voice quality. It is difficult to determine the extent of hypernasality, if at all present, because it is masked by the phonatory and articulation disorders. You may also observe that he attempts to occlude his nose on /t/ when he says "TV."

<u>Recommendations</u>: Treatment for the speech sound disorders is recommended. Treatment strategies would differ according to the error type and would be based on the phonetic/phonemic analysis. Compensatory errors would be treated via a phonetic motor learning approach (Ruscello & Vallino, 2014), while phonemic errors would be treated with phonemic-based strategies. A language assessment is also necessary for this patient. In addition, follow-up with the team otolaryngologist regarding the hoarse voice quality and voice therapy is recommended. Improvement in speech sound production and vocal quality will allow a better assessment of resonance balance.

Video Case Study 3.4.15

(*Note.* This child was 3.5 years old when he was presented in Audio 3.2.19. In this video, he is school aged.)

This is a 5-year-old male with repaired left unilateral cleft lip and palate who was internationally adopted at age 3. He first presented to the cleft palate team at age 3.5 years.

    This video includes this child's speech sample and his nasoendoscopic assessment of velopharyngeal function.

Case History

<u>Surgical</u>: Lip and palate repair completed by 1 year in birth country prior to adoption. OME treated with myringotomy and PE tubes.

<u>Dental</u>: Class I occlusion. Maxillary alveolar cleft with a very narrow oronasal fistula high in the vestibule.

<u>Hearing</u>: Responses to stimuli presented in sound field were within normal limits for at least the better ear. Otoscopy revealed tympanic membrane perforation in the right ear and PE tube in the left ear.

<u>Speech Therapy</u>: Enrolled in speech therapy to improve articulation

<u>Studies of Velopharyngeal Function</u>: Pressure-flow testing showed estimated velopharyngeal areas of 20.0 mm² on "hamper." There was complete overlap of oral pressure, nasal pressure, and nasal airflow during /-mp/ segments. In other words, the oral-nasal coupling was so complete that this child was unable to aerodynamically distinguish the /m/ from the /p/ segments in words. Estimated areas on /p/ in /papapa/ and /pipipi/ also exceeded 20 mm². Multiview videofluoroscopy showed a moderate to large gap with a coronal pattern of velopharyngeal movement.

Watch Video 3.4.15.

Speech Assessment:

Resonance: Moderate hypernasality

Nasal air emission: Audible nasal emission

Nasal grimace: Present during production of pressure sounds

Articulation: Developmental and obligatory errors

Phonation: WNL

Nasoendoscopic Assessment: Findings shows a moderate-sized circular velopharyngeal gap and good bilateral lateral pharyngeal wall movement.

Impression of Speech: The patient demonstrates nasal grimacing during the production of oral pressure sounds, and resonance quality is judged to be moderately hypernasal. Articulation produced within controlled contexts such as counting and sentence repetition is judged to be satisfactory in relation to chronological age, but note that the patient will sometimes front alveolars and palatal sounds. There is also a tendency for the patient to "overarticulate" sounds during the assessment. Note the shift in resonance when the nose is held. There is a notable change in articulation during spontaneous speech with reduced intelligibility. There is some inspiration during speech that can be heard. Audible nasal emission is present in the sample.

Recommendations: Speech therapy to focus on articulation and improve intelligibility. On the basis of perceptual and instrumental assessment findings, and in consultation with the surgeon, a pharyngoplasty is recommended to treat this child's VPD. This was discussed with the family, who indicated agreement to the procedure.

Video Case Study 3.4.16

(*Note.* This is the same child presented in Audio 3.3.18.)

This is a child with a repaired right unilateral cleft lip and palate who was internationally adopted at 32 months. In the first segment of this video, is 3.5 years old. In the second segment, he is 14 years old.

Case History

Surgical: Lip repair in this child's country of birth (date unknown). The palate was repaired at 33 months, 1 month after his arrival to this country. At age 6, he underwent sphincter pharyngoplasty to correct VPD and alveolar cleft repair at 9 years. Maxillary advancement will be done when he has reached skeletal maturity and completed facial growth. Myringotomies and PE tubes to treat OME were done at the time of palate repair with repeated sets of PE tubes several times thereafter during elementary school years.

Dental: Class I molar relationship at age 3.5 years. By 14 years of age, he developed a skeletal Class III malocclusion associated with maxillary hypoplasia.

Hearing: At the time of testing at 3.5 years of age, this child exhibited a mild conductive hearing loss in the left ear and normal hearing in the right ear. During his recent audiological testing at age 14, hearing was within normal limits, bilaterally.

Speech Therapy: Speech therapy initiated after palate repair and is enrolled in speech therapy at the time of this assessment. The focus of treatment was to achieve correct articulatory placement for oral consonants and eliminate compensatory errors associated with cleft palate. Articulation errors were all corrected but hypernasal speech persisted. Videonasoendoscopy confirmed the presence of a velopharyngeal gap for which surgery to correct VPD was recommended. He did not receive speech therapy after surgery to correct VPD.

Watch Video 3.4.16.

Note. In the first segment, this child is producing words from the Arizona Articulation Proficiency Scale-2. A list of the words he is producing is provided to facilitate your understanding (see below). He also produces a small conversational speech sample.

Words: telephone, cup, knife, ball, ring, shovel, banana, zipper (first try), zipper (second try with imitation), scissors, vacuum, watch, airplane, counting 1 to 5, 7.

Speech Assessment:

Parameters	Speech at 3.5 years old	Speech at 14 years old
Resonance	Mild hypernasality	Normal
Nasal air emission	Audible nasal emission on sibilants	None observed on mirror testing
Nasal grimace	Present during production of pressure sounds	Absent
Articulation	Glottal stops for oral stops, m/k substitution in "cup," but the patient produces the /b/ in "ball" correctly	Very slight inconsistent distortion on /r/ Very slight oral distortions on sibilants
Phonation	Hoarse vocal quality with laryngeal tension, hard glottal attack	WNL

Impression of Speech: At age 3.5, this child's speech is judged to be mildly hypernasal and there is also mild hoarseness with laryngeal tension that results in hard glottal attack. Note that during the production of pressure sounds, there are instances of nasal grimace, glottal stops for oral stops, audible nasal air emission on sibilants, and m/k substitution in "cup," but the patient produces the /b/ in "ball" correctly. At age 14, resonance is judged to be within normal limits. His oral distortions are a consequence of the malocclusion, which will be corrected in the future. These errors and that of the very slight inconsistent distortion on /r/ would most likely be imperceptible to the untrained listener. He is easy to understand.

Recommendations at Age 3.5: Speech therapy to correct the compensatory speech errors and incorporate discrimination and production drills directed to the hard glottal attack. Continual monitoring through the cleft palate clinic to include imaging of the velopharyngeal valving mechanism when he produces oral consonants more consistently in order to assess optimal function of the mechanism during speech. Follow-up with the team otolaryngologist regarding the hoarse voice quality and voice therapy is recommended.

Recommendations of Age 14: The combined effects of speech therapy and surgery to correct VPD resulted in speech that is well within functional limits. There are no specific recommendations for additional intervention.

Video Case Study 3.4.17

(*Note.* Before and after insertion of speech appliance to correct VPD.)

This is a 10-year-old female with Pierre Robin sequence and a repaired cleft of the soft palate. She presented with hypernasal speech and compensatory speech sound errors. Parents were not interested in a surgical option but wanted a prosthesis fabricated for the patient, which was done. In the first segment of the video, you will hear this child's speech without the palatal appliance. In the following segment, you will have the opportunity to hear her speech while wearing the palatal appliance.

Case History

Surgical: The palatal defect was repaired at 12 months and a fistula developed, which was later surgically closed.

Dental: Dentition is within normal limits.

Hearing: At the time of testing, hearing was within normal limits, bilaterally.

Speech Therapy: She presented with hypernasality and compensatory speech sound errors. She did receive treatment for the compensatory errors.

Studies of Velopharyngeal Function: Pressure-flow studies showed reduced oral pressure in the presence of concomitant nasal air pressure and airflow. Videonasoendoscopy showed a coronal pattern of velopharyngeal movement without complete closure.

 Watch Video 3.4.17.

Speech Assessment:

Parameters	Before speech appliance	After speech applicance
Resonance	Moderate hypernasality	Normal resonance balance
Nasal air emission	NA	NA
Nasal grimace	Not observed	Not observed
Articulation	Compensatory errors	Correct oral placement
Phonation	WNL	WNL

Impression of Speech Before and After Speech Applicance: This patient had undergone successful speech therapy to correct compensatory speech errors, but the VPD prevented the generation of satisfactory oral pressure for plosives, fricatives, and affricates. In addition, resonance quality remained hypernasal. The patient's parents did not want additional surgery, so they opted for the fabrication of a palatal prosthesis. After insertion of the appliance, note that resonance is WNL and the patient can generate adequate oral pressure in the presence of correct oral placements for the pressure sounds. Phonation is satisfactory. The appliance was effective in improving speech and resonance.

Recommendations: Continued wear of the speech appliance is supported and periodic monitoring via the cleft palate clinic.

Video Case Study 3.4.18

(*Note.* Before and after surgery to correct VPD.)

This is an 8.5-year-old male with repaired isolated cleft of the secondary palate who first presented to the cleft palate team at age 3 years. Speech assessments over the course of subsequent team visits suggested gradual changes in resonance, confirmed using pressure-flow studies. In this video, you will have the opportunity to follow this child through the course of his treatment. In Part 1, you will hear him when he is 5 years old and receiving speech therapy. In Part 2, he is 8 years old. You hear a sample of his speech followed by his nasoendoscopic assessment. In Part 3, you will hear his speech 9 weeks after surgery to correct VPD.

Case History

Surgical: Palate repair at 9 months of age. Myringotomies and PE tubes to treat OME at the time of palate repair. Pushback revision palatoplasty with buccal flaps at age 8.5 years to correct VPD.

Dental: Class I occlusion incisal relationship and molar relationship; slight crossbite on left side

Hearing: At the time of testing, hearing was within normal limits, bilaterally.

Speech Therapy: He has a history of speech therapy to correct articulation errors. At age 5 years, he was enrolled in speech therapy to improve articulation for /s, z, ʃ, tʃ/ and continued to receive this service throughout the course of his treatment.

Preoperative Studies of Velopharyngeal Function: Pressure-flow testing indicated inadequate velopharyngeal closure as evidenced by nasal airflow exceeding 106 mL/s during /pi/ (normed range for age; 5.1–13.3). Multiview videofluoroscopy showed incomplete velar closure and minimal lateral pharyngeal wall movement resulting in a coronal pattern of velopharyngeal closure. Instrumental assessment findings confirmed VPD, for which surgery was recommended.

<u>Postoperative Studies of Velopharyngeal Function at 9 Weeks</u>:
Pressure-flow testing showed a change in velopharyngeal
function as evidenced by a reduction in nasal airflow rates
that ranged from 15 to 24 mL/s during /pi/.

Watch Video 3.4.18.

<u>Speech Assessment</u>:

Parameters	Enrolled in speech therapy, 5 years old	Before surgery to correct VPD, 8 years old	9 weeks after surgery, 8.5 years old
Resonance	Moderate hypernasality	Mild to moderate hypernasality	WNL
Nasal air emission	Nasal turbulence on "five" and "six"		No audible nasal air emission perceived
Nasal grimace	Present	Present	None perceived
Articulation	Posterior nasal fricative, a maladaptive articulation error Of note, the presence of the posterior nasal fricative was confirmed	Maladaptive errors corrected with treatment; articulation placement is appropriate	Accurate articulation placement

Parameters	Enrolled in speech therapy, 5 years old	Before surgery to correct VPD, 8 years old	9 weeks after surgery, 8.5 years old
Articulation *continued*	during the clinical assessment when the clinician occluded his nose, upon which he actively produced an oral stop and no frication for the sibilant.		
Phonation	WNL		WNL

<u>Nasoendoscopic Assessment (Before Treatment)</u>: There is limited movement of both the velum and lateral pharyngeal walls with an elliptical opening (coronal pattern) that appears continuous during the production of oral speech items. Bubbling can be observed throughout the assessment. Occasionally, there is touch closure of the right side.

<u>Impression of Speech at the Different Time Intervals</u>: Before speech therapy, this child presented with anterior nasal frication on sibilants and moderate hypernasality. There was also an instance of nasal turbulence. The focus of speech therapy was to eliminate this maladaptive error pattern. Therapy was successful, but the hypernasality persisted, which is expected since there is a velopharyngeal deficit. Articulation placement was appropriate. A speech assessment conducted 3 weeks after surgery suggested adequate velopharyngeal function. Although findings appear to be positive in that the hypernasality is ameliorated, continued monitoring of this child's

speech closely over the course of the year is needed to determine a more definitive effect of treatment.

Recommendations: Continue routine monitoring of resonance and velopharyngeal function, including pressure-flow studies over time with routine follow-up by the cleft palate team. There are no specific recommendations for speech therapy.

Video Case Study 3.4.19

(*Note.* Before and after surgery to improve velopharyngeal function.)

This final video is that of a 10-year-old female with congenital ectodermal dysplasia, as part of Bartsocas Papas syndrome (BPS) and bilateral cleft lip and palate. She is shown during her course of treatment for VPD. In the first segment of the video, she is 5 years old, during which time she was enrolled in speech. In the second segment, she is 10 years old, when she was seen 3 months after surgery to correct VPD.

Case History

Medical: Born at 34 weeks. Very protrusive premaxilla deviated to the left side and underdeveloped soft palate musculature. Recurrent episodes of OME. History of obstructive sleep apnea (OSA).

Surgical:

■   8 weeks: Presurgical palatal appliance
■   4 months: Appliance was removed and a bilateral lip adhesion was done.
■   7 months: Definitive lip repair at 7 months
■   11 months: Palate repair and myringotomy and PE tubes at the time of palate repair to manage OME (note: PE tubes were replaced three times, thereafter)
■   4 years: Pushback revision palatoplasty with buccal flaps to correct VPD
■   8 years: Maxillary alveolar cleft repair
■   9.9 years: VPD persisted after the pushback revision procedure. After this, the child was reevaluated for OSA and considered to no longer be at risk for the condition, and a sphincter pharyngoplasty was done to correct VPD.

Dental: Class III with posterior crossbite

Hearing: At the time of testing, hearing within normal limits, bilaterally

<u>Speech Therapy</u>: Early history of speech therapy to correct compensatory articulation errors associated with VPD

<u>Studies of Velopharyngeal Function</u>: Imaging of the velopharyngeal port using both multiview videofluoroscopy and videonasoendoscopy was done at age 9. Findings showed incomplete velar closure and minimal lateral pharyngeal wall movement, resulting in a coronal pattern of velopharyngeal closure. Instrumental findings confirm the presence of VPD. Based upon these results, a sphincter pharyngoplasty was recommended.

> ## *Watch Video 3.4.19.*

<u>Speech Assessment</u>:

Parameters	Receiving speech therapy, 5 years old	3 months postsurgery, 10 years old
Resonance	Moderate hypernasality	Mild hyponasality
Nasal air emission	Present on mirror test	
Nasal grimace	Inconsistent and slight	None
Articulation	Compensatory and developmental errors	Good articulation
Phonation	Mild hoarseness	Unremarkable

<u>Impression of Speech Before and After Surgery</u>: At age 5, speech was marked by moderate hypernasality. There was d/ dʒ in "jam," glottal stop on /g/ in "buggy," but good bilabial production of /p/ and /b/. She did not produce /s/. Hard glottal

attack on vowels during /pa pa pa/. After surgery, resonance is mildly hyponasal, as often is the case when a pharyngeal flap is done. Phonation is unremarkable. Note that despite her dental and occlusal anomalies, she has very good articulation.

Recommendations: Continue follow-up with the cleft palate team for care. Monitor hyponasality and any additional needs that are related to the cleft.

References

American Cleft Palate–Craniofacial Association. (n.d.). *Speech samples.* Retrieved from http://www.acpa-cpf.org/education/educational _resources/speech_samples/

American Cleft Palate–Craniofacial Association (2018). *Parameters for the evaluation and treatment of patients with cleft lip/palate or other craniofacial anomalies.* Retrieved from http://www.acpa-cpf.org/standardscat/parameters-of-care

American Speech-Language-Hearing Association. (n.d.-b). *Cleft lip and palate.* Retrieved from http://www.asha.org/Practice-Portal/ Clinical-Topics/Cleft-Lip-and-Palate

American Speech-Language-Hearing Association. (2012). *2012 Schools survey. Survey summary report: Number and type of responses, SLPs.* Retrieved from http://www.asha.org

American Speech-Language-Hearing Association. (n.d.-a). *Cultural competence.* (Pratical Portal). Retrieved from http://www. asha.org/Practice-Portal/Professional-Issues/Cultural-Competence/. Retrieved from http://www.asha.org/Practice-Portal/ Professional-Issues/Cultural-Competence

Bankson, N. W., & Bernthal, J. E. (2004). Phonological assessment procedures. *Articulation and phonological disorders* (5th ed.). Boston, MA: Pearson Allyn Bacon.

Bedwinek, A. P. (2007). *An analysis of nees: School speech-language pathologists and children born with cleft lip/palate* (Unpublished doctoral dissertation). Union University, Jackson TN.

Bedwinek, A. P., Kummer, A. W., Rice, G. B., & Grames, L. M. (2010). Current training and continuing education needs of preschool and school-based speech-language pathologists regarding children with cleft lip/palate. *Language, Speech, and Hearing Services in Schools, 41,* 405–414.

Bell-Berti, F. (1993). Understanding velic motor control: Studies of segmental context. In M. K. Huffman & R. A. Krakow (Eds.), *Phonetics and phonology: Vol. 5. Nasals, nasalization, and the velum* (pp. 63–86). San Diego, CA: Academic Press.

Bernthal, J. E., Bankson, N. W., & Flipsen, P. (2017). *Articulation and phonological disorders: speech sound disorders in patients* (8th ed.). Boston, MA: Pearson Education.

Bessell, A., Sell, D., Whiting, P., Roulstone, S., Albery, L., & Persson, M. (2013). Speech and language therapy interventions for children with cleft palate: A systematic review. *The Cleft Palate-Craniofacial Journal, 50*, e1–e17.

Byiers, B. J., Reichle, J., & Symons, F. J. (2012). Single-subject experimental design for evidence-based practice. *American Journal of Speech-Language Pathology, 21*, 397–414.

Cavalli, L. (2011). Voice assessment and intervention. In S. Howard & A. Lohmander (Eds.), *Cleft palate speech: Assessment and intervention* (pp. 181–198). Hoboken, NJ: Wiley.

Chapman, K. (1993). Phonologic processes in children with cleft palate. *The Cleft Palate-Craniofacial Journal, 30*, 64–71.

Chapman, K. (2009). Speech and language of children with cleft palate: Interactions and influences. In K. T. Moller & L. E. Glaze (Eds.), *Cleft lip and palate: Interdisciplinary issues and treatment* (2nd ed., pp. 243–292). Austin, TX: Pro-Ed.

Chapman, K. L., & Hardin, M. A. (1992). Phonetic and phonological skills of two-year-olds with cleft palate. *The Cleft Palate–Craniofacial Journal, 29*, 435–443.

Cheng, L. R. L. (1990). Asian-American cultural perspectives on birth defects: Focus on cleft palate. *The Cleft Palate–Craniofacial Journal, 27*, 294–300.

Choi, B. C., & Pak, A. W. (2006). Multidisciplinarity, interdisciplinarity and transdisciplinarity in health research, services, education and policy: 1. Definitions, objectives, and evidence of effectiveness. *Clinical and Investigative Medicine, 29*, 351–364.

Cleft Palate Foundation. (n.d.) *U.S. team listing.* Retrieved from http://www.cleftline.org/parents-individuals/team-care/

Cohn, E. (2013, June 6). On the pulse: Combining strengths in craniofacial treatment: Cleft palate and craniofacial teams provide a long-established model of interprofessional care. *The ASHA Leader, 18*, 30–31.

Croneberger, R., Jr., & Luck, C. (1975). Defining information and referral service. *Library Journal, 100*, 1984–1987.

Dailey, S., & Wilson, K. (2015). Communicating with a cleft palate team: Improving coordination of care across treatment settings. *SIG 5 Perspectives on Speech Science and Orofacial Disorders, 25*, 35–38.

Dalston, R. M., Martinkosky, S. J., & Hinton, V. A. (1987). Stuttering prevalence among patients at risk for velopharyngeal inadequacy: A preliminary investigation. *The Cleft Palate Journal, 24*, 233–239.

D'Antonio, L., & Scherer, N. J. (2008). Communication disorders associated with cleft palate. In J.E. Losee & R. E. Kirschner (Eds.), *Comprehensive cleft care* (pp. 114–135). New York, NY: McGraw-Hill.

D'Antonio, L. L., Muntz, H., Providence, M., & Marsh, J. (1988). Laryngeal/voice findings in patients with velopharyngeal dysfunction. *Laryngoscope, 98*, 432–438.

Dickson, D. R., & Maue-Dickson, W. (1982). *Anatomical and physiological bases of speech*. Boston, MA: Little, Brown.

Dobblesteyn, C., Kay-Raining Bird, E., Parker, J., Griffiths, C., Budden, A., & Flood, K. (2014). Effectiveness of corrective babbling speech treatment program for patients with a history of cleft palate or velopharyngeal dysfunction. *The Cleft Palate–Craniofacial Journal, 51*, 129–144.

Edwards, N., Davies, B., Ploeg, J., Virani, T., & Skelly, J. (2007). Implementing nursing best practice guidelines: Impact on patient referrals. *BMC Nursing, 6*, 4.

Elbert, M., & Gierut, J. (1986). *Handbook of clinical phonology*. San Diego, CA: College-Hill Press.

Esghi, M., Baylis, A., Vallino, L. D., Crais, N., Preisser, J., Vivaldi, D., Dorry, J., & Zajac, D. J. (2017). *Lexical and morphosyntactic abilities in two-year-old children with and without cleft palate*. Paper presented at the Annual Meeting of the American Cleft Palate-Craniofacial Association, Colorado Springs, CO.

Eshghi, M., Dorry, J., Crais, E., Baylis, A., Vallino, L., Vivaldi, D., . . . Zajac, D. J. (2017, March). *Development of symbolic behavior in children with and without repaired cleft palate*. Poster presented at the Annual Meeting of the American Cleft Palate–Craniofacial Association, Colorado Springs, CO.

Eshghi, M., Zajac, D. J., Bijankhan, M., & Shirazi, M. (2013). Spectral analysis of word-initial alveolar and velar plosives produced by Iranian children with cleft lip and palate. *Clinical Linguistics & Phonetics, 27*, 213–219.

Fletcher, S. G. (1972). Contingencies for bioelectric modification of nasality. *Journal of Speech and Hearing Disorders, 37*, 329–346.

Folkins, J. D. (1988). Velopharyngeal nomenclature. Incompetence, inadequacy, insufficiency and dysfunction. *Cleft Palate Journal, 25*, 413–416.

Foot, C., Naylor, C., & Imison, C. (2010). *The quality of GP diagnosis and referral*. Retrieved July 29, 2017, from https://www.kings fund.org.uk/projects/gp-inquiry/diagnosis-referral

Fudala, J. B., & Reynolds, W. M. (2000). *Arizona Articulation Proficiency Scale* (3rd ed.). Austin, TX: Pro-Ed.

Gibbon, F. E., & Crampin, L. (2001). An electropalatographic investigation of middorsum palatal stops in an adult with repaired cleft palate. *Cleft Palate–Craniofacial Journal, 38*, 96–105.

Gibbon, F. E., Ellis, L., & Crampin, L. (2004). Articulatory placement for /t/, /d/, /k/ and /g/ targets in school age children with speech disorders associated with cleft palate. *Clinical Linguistics & Phonetics, 18*, 391–404.

Gilleard, O., Sell, D., Ghanem, A. M., Tavsanoglu, Y., Birch, M., & Sommerlad, B. (2014). Submucous cleft palate: A systematic review of surgical management based on perceptual and instrumental analysis. *The Cleft Palate–Craniofacial Journal, 51*, 686–695.

Glaze, L. (2009). Behavioral approaches to treating velopharyngeal dysfunction and nasality. In K. T. Moller & L. E. Glaze (Eds.), *Cleft lip and palate: Interdisciplinary issues and treatment.* Austin, TX: Pro-Ed.

Golding-Kushner, K. J. (1995). Treatment of articulation and resonance disorders associated with cleft palate and VPI. In R. J. Shprintzen & J. Bardach (Eds.), *Cleft palate speech management: A multidisciplinary approach* (pp. 327–351). St. Louis, MO: Mosby.

Golding-Kushner, K. J. (2001). *Therapy techniques for cleft palate speech and related disorders.* San Diego, CA: Singular.

Golding-Kushner, K. J., & Shprintzen, R. J. (2011). *Velo-cardio-facial syndrome: Vol. II. Treatment of communication disorders.* San Diego, CA: Plural.

Goldman, R., & Fristoe, M. (2015). *Goldman-Fristoe Test of Articulation-3.* San Antonio, TX: Pearson.

Gorlin, R. J., & Baylis, A. L. (2009). Developmental and genetic aspects of cleft lip and palate. In K. T. Moller & L. E. Glaze (Eds.) *Interdisciplinary management of cleft lip and palate: For clinicians by clinicians* (pp. 103–169). Austin, TX: Pro-Ed.

Grames, L. M. (2004). Implementing treatment recommendations: Role of the craniofacial team speech-language pathologist in working with the client's speech-language pathologist. *SIG 5 Perspectives on Speech Science and Orofacial Disorders, 14*, 6–9.

Grames, L. M. (2008). Advancing into the 21st century: Care for individuals with cleft palate or craniofacial differences. *The ASHA Leader, 13*, 10–12.

Grames, L. M., & Stahl, M. H. (2017). An innovative collaborative treatment model: The community-based speech-language pathologist and cleft palate team. *The Cleft Palate-Craniofacial Journal, 54*, 242–244.

Hardin-Jones, M. A., & Chapman, K. I. (2015, April). *The significance of nasal substitutions in the early phonology of toddlers with repaired cleft palate.* Poster presented at the Annual Meeting of the American Cleft Palate–Craniofacial Association, Palm Springs, CA.

Hardin-Jones, M., Chapman, K., & Scherer, N. J. (2006). Early intervention in children with cleft palate. *The ASHA Leader, 11*, 8–32.

Harding, A., & Grunwell, P. (1998). Notes and discussion active versus passive cleft-type speech characteristics. *International Journal of Language & Communication Disorders, 33*, 329–352.

Health Insurance Portability and Accountability Act of 1996 (HIPAA). Public Law 104-191, 104th Congress.

Henningsson, G., Kuehn, D. P., Sell, D., Sweeny, T., Trost-Cardamone, J. E., & Whitehill, T. L. (2008). Universal parameters for reporting speech outcomes in individuals with cleft palate. *The Cleft Palate–Craniofacial Journal, 45*, 1–17.

Henningsson, G. E., & Isberg, A. M. (1986). Velopharyngeal movements in patients alternating between oral and glottal articulation: A clinical and cineradiographical study. *The Cleft Palate Journal, 23*, 1–9.

Hixon, T. J., Weismer, G., & Hoit, J. D. (2008). *Preclinical speech science: Anatomy physiology acoustics perception.* San Diego, CA: Plural.

John, A., Sell, D., Sweeney, T., Harding-Bell, A., & Williams, A. (2006). The cleft audit protocol for speech—augmented: A validated and reliable measure for auditing cleft speech. *The Cleft Palate–Craniofacial Journal, 43*, 272–288.

Justice, L. M., & Fey, M. E. (2004, September 9). Evidence-based practice in schools: Integrating craft and theory with science and data. *ASHA Leader, 9*, 4–32.

Karnell, M. P., Bailey, P., Johnson, L., Dragan, A., & Canady, J. W. (2005). Facilitating communication among speech pathologists treating children with cleft palate. *The Cleft Palate–Craniofacial Journal, 42*, 585–588.

Kent, R. D. (1988). Prosody in the young child. In D. E. Yoder & R. D. Kent (Eds.), *Decision making in speech-language pathology* (pp. 144–145). Philadelphia, PA: B. C. Decker.

Kent, R. D., Miolo, G., & Bloedel, S. (1994). The intelligibility of children's speech: A review of evaluation procedures. *American Journal of Speech-Language Pathology, 3*, 81–95.

Klein, J. T. (1990). *Interdisciplinarity: History, theory, and practice.* Detroit, MI: Wayne State University Press.

Kummer, A. W. (2001). Speech therapy for effects of velopharyngeal dysfunction. In A. W. Kummer (Ed.), *Cleft palate and craniofacial anomalies: The effects of speech and resonance* (pp. 459–482). San Diego, CA: Singular.

Kummer, A. W. (2008). Speech therapy for effects of velopharyngeal dysfunction. In A. W. Kummer (Ed.), *Cleft palate and craniofacial anomalies: The effects of speech and resonance* (2nd ed., p. 300). San Diego, CA: Singular.

Kummer, A. (2014). *Cleft palate and craniofacial anomalies: Effects on speech and resonance* (3rd ed.). Clifton Park, NY: Cengage Learning.

Kuster, J. M. (2010, December). Resources for clients with craniofacial abnormalities. *The ASHA Leader, 15.*

LeDuc, J. A. (2008). Cleft palate and/or velopharyngeal dysfunction: Assessment and treatment. *SIG 16 Perspectives on School-Based Issues, 9,* 155–161.

Linking to other services: Referral guidelines for family relationship centres and the family relationship advice line. (n.d.). Retrieved from https://www.ag.gov.au/FamiliesAndMarriage/Families/FamilyRelationshipServices/Documents/Referral%20Guidelines.pdf

Lof, G. L., & Ruscello, D. (2013). Don't blow this therapy session! *Perspectives on Speech Science and Orofacial Disorders, 23,* 38–48.

Lorenz, A. D., Mauksch, L. B., & Gawinski, B. A. (1999). Models of collaboration. *Primary Care, 2,* 401–410.

Lubker, J. F. (1975). Normal velopharyngeal function in speech. *Clinics in Plastic Surgery, 2,* 249–259.

Marino, V. C. C., Williams, W. N., Wharton, P. W., Paulk, M. F., Dutka-Souza, J. C. R., & Schulz, G. M. (2005). Immediate and sustained changes in tongue movement with an experimental palatal "fistula": A case study. *The Cleft Palate-Craniofacial Journal, 42,* 286–296.

McCauley, R. J., Strand, E., Lof, G. L., Schooling, T., & Frymark, T. (2009). Evidence-based systematic review: Effects of nonspeech oral motor exercises on speech. *American Journal of Speech-Language Pathology, 18,* 343–360.

McWilliams, B. J. (1982). Cleft palate. In G. H. Shames & E. H. Wiig (Eds.), *Human communication disorders: An introduction* (pp. 330–369). Columbus, OH: Merrill.

McWilliams, B. J., Bluestone, C. D., & Musgrave, R. H. (1969). Diagnostic implications of vocal cord nodules in children with cleft palate. *Laryngoscope, 79,* 2072–2080.

McWilliams, B. J., Glaser, E. R., Philips, B. J., Lawrence, C., Lavorato, A. S., Beery, Q. C., & Skolnick, M. L. (1981). A comparative study of four methods of evaluating velopharyngeal adequacy. *Plastic and Reconstructive Surgery, 68*(1), 1–9.

McWilliams, B. J., Morris, H. L., & Shelton, R. L. (1984). Articulation and intelligibility. *Cleft palate speech,* 232–255. Philadelphia, PA: B. C. Decker.

McWilliams, B. J., Morris, H. L., & Shelton, R. L. (1990). *Cleft palate speech* (2nd ed.). Philadelphia, PA: B. C. Decker.

McWilliams, B. J., & Philips, B. J. (1979). *Audio seminars in speech pathology: Velopharyngeal incompetence.* Toronto, Canada: B. C. Decker.

Marsh, J. L., Vig, K. W., & Bumsted, R. M. (1988). Minimal standards for reporting the results of surgery on patients with cleft lip, cleft palate, or both: A proposal. *The Cleft Palate Journal, 25,* 3–7.

Meyerson, M. D. (1990). Cultural considerations in the treatment of Latinos with craniofacial malformations. *The Cleft Palate–Craniofacial Journal, 27,* 279–288.

Milenkovic, P. (2000). *TF32* [Software]. Madison, WI: University of Wisconsin.

Moller, K. T. (1994). Dental-occlusal and other oral conditions and speech. In J. Bernthal & N. Bankson (Eds.), *Child phonology: Characteristics, assessment, and intervention with special populations* (pp. 3–28). New York, NY: Thieme Medical.

Moon, J. B., Smith, A. E., Folkins, J. W., Lemke, J. H., & Gartlan, M. (1994). Coordination of velopharyngeal muscle activity during positioning of the soft palate. *The Cleft Palate–Craniofacial Journal, 31,* 45–55.

Moore, E. (2016). Special considerations for evaluation and treatment of Spanish-speaking patients with cleft palate. *Perspectives of the ASHA Special Interest Groups, SIG 5, 1*(2), 41–49.

Morgan, A., O'Gara, M., Albert, M., & Kapp-Simon, K. (2016). Clinical decision making for the internationally adopted patient with cleft lip and palate. *Perspectives of the ASHA Special Interest Groups, SIG 5, 1*(2), 27–39.

Morley, M. E. (1970). *Cleft palate and speech* (7th ed.). Edinburgh, UK: Churchill Livingstone.

Morris, H. L. (1992). Some questions and answers about velopharyngeal dysfunction during speech. *American Journal of Speech-Language Pathology, 1,* 26–28.

Nancarrow, S. A., Booth, A., Ariss, S., Smith, T., Enderby, P., & Roots, A. (2013). Ten principles of good interdisciplinary team work. *Human Resources for Health, 11,* 19.

Napoli, J. A., & Vallino, L. D. (2017). Maxillary advancement. In D. J. Zajac & L. D. Vallino (Eds.), *Evaluation and management of cleft lip and palate.* San Diego, CA: Plural.

Nester, J. (2016). The importance of interprofessional practice and education in the era of accountable care. *North Carolina Medical Journal, 77,* 128–132.

Okazaki, K., Kato, M., & Onizuka, T. (1991). Palate morphology in children with cleft palate with palatalized articulation. *Annals of Plastic Surgery, 26,* 156–163.

Pamplona, M., & Ysunza, A. (1999). A comparative trial of two modalities of speech intervention for cleft palate children: Phonologic vs. articulatory approach. *International Journal of Pediatric Otorhinolaryngology, 49,* 2–27.

Peterson, S. J. (1975). Nasal emission as a component of the misarticulation of sibilants and affricates. *Journal of Speech and Hearing Disorders, 40,* 106–114.

Peterson-Falzone, S. J. (1995). Speech outcomes in adolescents with cleft lip and palate. *The Cleft Palate–Craniofacial Journal, 32,* 125–128.

Peterson-Falzone, S. J., & Graham, M. S. (1990). Phoneme-specific nasal emission in children with and without physical anomalies of the velopharyngeal mechanism. *Journal of Speech and Hearing Disorders, 55,* 132–139.

Peterson-Falzone, S. J., Hardin-Jones, M. A., & Karnell, M. (2001). *Cleft palate speech* (3rd ed.). St. Louis, MO: Mosby.

Peterson-Falzone, S. J., Hardin-Jones, M. A., & Karnell, M. (2010). *Cleft palate speech* (4th ed.). St. Louis, MO: Mosby.

Peterson-Falzone, S. J., Trost-Cardamone, J. E., Karnell, M., & Hardin-Jones, M. A. (2006). *Treating cleft palate speech.* St. Louis, MO: Mosby.

Peterson-Falzone, S. J., Trost-Cardamone, J. E., Karnell, M., & Hardin-Jones, M. A. (2017). *Treating cleft palate speech* (2nd ed.). St. Louis, MO: Mosby.

Proctor, D. F. (1982). The upper airway. In D. F. Proctor & I. B. Anderson (Eds.), *The nose: Upper airway physiology and the atmospheric environment.* New York: Elsevier Biomedical Press.

Riski, J. E. (1995). Speech assessment of adolescents. *The Cleft Palate–Craniofacial Journal, 32,* 109–113.

Riski, J. E. (2003). Improving your clinical competence with unique articulation disorders. Retrieved from http//www.choa.org./craniofacial/speech-3.shtml

Rood, S. R., & Doyle, W. J. (1978). Morphology of tensor veli palatini, tensor tympani, and dilatator tubae muscles. *Annals of Otology, Rhinology & Laryngology, 87*(2), 202–210.

Ruscello, D. M. (1993). A motor skill learning treatment program for sound system disorders, *Seminars in Speech and Language, 14,* 106–118.

Ruscello, D. M. (2004). Considerations for behavioral treatment of velopharyngeal closure for speech. In K. Bzoch (Ed.), *Communicative disorders related to cleft lip and palate* (5th ed.). Austin, TX: Pro-Ed.

Ruscello, D. M. (2008a). *Treating articulation and phonological disorders in children.* St. Louis, MO: Mosby Elsevier.

Ruscello, D. M. (2008b). An examination of non-speech oral motor exercises for children with VPI. *Seminars in Speech and Language, 29,* 294–303.

Ruscello, D. M. (2017). School-based intervention. In D. Zajac & L. Vallino (Eds.), *Evaluation and management of cleft lip and palate.* San Diego, CA: Plural.

Ruscello, D. M., Tekieli, M. E., & Van Sickels, J. E. (1985). Speech production before and after orthognathic surgery: A review. *Oral Surgery, Oral Medicine, and Oral Pathology, 59,* 10–14.

Ruscello, D. M., & Vallino, L. (2014). The application of motor learning concepts to the treatment of children with compensatory speech sound errors. *Perspectives on Speech Science and Orofacial Disorders American Speech-Language-Hearing Association (ASHA Perspectives content).* Retrieved from http://journals.asha.org/perspectives/terms.dtl

Ruscello, D., Yanero, D., & Ghalichebaf, M. (1995). Cooperative service delivery between a university clinic and a school system. *Language, Speech, and Hearing Services in Schools, 26,* 273–276.

Rvachew, S., & Brosseau-Lapre, F. (2018). *Developmental phonological disorders* (2nd ed.). San Diego, CA: Plural.

Santelmann, I., Sussman, J., & Chapman, K. (1999). Perception of mid-dorsum palatal stops from the speech of three children with repaired cleft palate. *The Cleft Palate–Craniofacial Journal, 36,* 233–241.

Scherer, N. J. (2017). Early linguistic development and intervention. In D. J. Zajac & L. D. Vallino (Eds.), *Evaluation and management of cleft lip and palate.* San Diego, CA: Plural.

Scherer, N. J., D'antonio, L. L., & McGahey, H. (2008). Early intervention for speech impairment in children with cleft palate. *The Cleft Palate–Craniofacial Journal, 45,* 18–31.

Scherer, N. J., & Kaiser, A. (2007). Early intervention in children with cleft palate. *Infants and Young Children, 20,* 355–366.

See-Scape (1986). Austin, TX: Pro-Ed.

Sell, D., Harding, A., & Grunwell, P. (1994). A screening assessment of cleft palate speech (Great Ormond Street Speech Assessment). *International Journal of Language & Communication Disorders, 29,* 1–15.

Sell, D., Harding, A., & Grunwell, P. (1999). GOS. SP. ASS.'98: an assessment for speech disorders associated with cleft palate and/or velopharyngeal dysfunction (revised). *International Journal of Language & Communication Disorders, 34,* 17–33.

Shelton, R. L., & Trier, W. C. (1976). Issues involved in the evaluation of velopharyngeal closure. *The Cleft Palate Journal, 13,* 127–137.

Shprintzen, R. J. (2000). *Syndrome identification for speech-language pathology.* San Diego, CA: Singular.

Shriberg, L. D., Kent, R. D., Karlsson, H. B., McSweeny, J. L., Nadler, C. J., & Brown, R. L. (2003). A diagnostic marker for speech delay associated with otitis media with effusion: Backing of obstruents. *Clinical Linguistics & Phonetics, 17,* 529–547.

Skahan, S. M., Watson, M., & Lof, G. L. (2007). Speech-language pathologists' assessment practices for children with suspected speech sound disorders: Results of a national survey. *American Journal of Speech-Language Pathology, 16,* 246–259.

Skolnick, M. L., McCall, G. N., & Barnes, M. (1972). The sphincteric mechanism of velopharyngeal closure. *The Cleft Palate Journal, 10,* 286–305.

St. Louis, K. O., Ruscello, D. M., & Lass, N. J. (1991). Coexistence of communication disorders: Implications for clinical training. *National Student Speech Language Hearing Association Journal, 18,* 146–150.

Swift, J. Q. (2009). Oral and maxillofacial surgery: Management of the alveolar cleft and jaw discrepancies. In K. T. Moller & L. E. Glaze (Eds.), *Cleft lip and palate: Interdisciplinary issues and treatment* (2nd ed., pp. 573–600). Austin, TX: Pro-Ed.

Symonds, K., & Zajac, D. J. (2009, November). *Acoustic characteristics of posterior nasal fricatives: Evidence for oral stops.* Paper presented at the ASHA Convention, New Orleans, LA.

Templin, M. C., & Darley, F. L. (1969). *The Templin-Darley Tests of Articulation.* Iowa City, IA: University of Iowa Bureau of Educational Research and Service.

Toliver-Weddington, G. (1990). Cultural considerations in the treatment of craniofacial malformations in African Americans. *The Cleft Palate–Craniofacial Journal, 27,* 289–293.

Tomes, L. A., Kuehn, D. P., & Peterson-Falzone, S. J. (2004). Research considerations for behavioral treatments of velopharyngeal impairment. In K. Bzoch (Ed.), *Communicative disorders related to cleft lip and palate* (5th ed., pp. 797–846). Austin, TX: Pro-Ed.

Torres, I. G. (2013, February 1). Know what you don't know. *The ASHA Leader, 18,* 38–41.

Tortora, C., Meazzini, M. C., Garattini, G., & Brusati, R. (2008). Prevalence of abnormalities in dental structure, position, and eruption pattern in a population of unilateral and bilateral cleft lip and palate patients. *The Cleft Palate–Craniofacial Journal, 45,* 154–162.

Treatment Improvement Protocol (TIP) Series. (2014). *Chapter 5: Effective referrals and collaborations. Integrating Substance Abuse Treatment and Vocational Service.* U.S. Department of Health and Human Services, Center for 91-99. Retrieved from http://store .samhsa.gov/shin/content/SMA12-4216/SMA12-4216.pdf

Trost, J. E. (1981). Articulatory additions to the description of the speech of persons with cleft palate. *The Cleft Palate Journal, 18,* 193–203.

Trost-Cardamone, J. E. (1990a). The development of speech: Assessing cleft palate misarticulations. In D. A. Kernahan & S. W. Rosenstein (Eds.), *Cleft lip and palate* (pp. 225–235). Baltimore, MD: Williams & Wilkins.

Trost-Cardamone, J. E. (1990b). Speech: Anatomy, physiology, and pathology. In D. A. Kernahan & S. W. Rosenstein (Eds.), *Cleft lip and palate* (pp. 91–103). Baltimore, MD: Williams & Wilkins.

Trost-Cardamone, J. E. (2009). Articulation and phonologic assessment procedures and treatment decisions. In K. T. Moller & L. E. Glaze (Eds.), *Cleft lip and palate: Interdisciplinary issues and treatment* (2nd ed., pp. 377–414). Austin, TX: Pro-Ed.

Trost-Cardamone, J. E. (2013). *Cleft palate speech.* Rockville, MD: ASHA Product Sales.

Trost-Cardamone, J. E., & Bernthal, J. E. (1993). Articulation assessment procedures and treatment decisions. In K. T. Moller & C. D. Starr (Eds.), *Cleft palate: Interdisciplinary issues and treatment* (pp. 307–336). Austin, TX: Pro-Ed.

Vallino, L. D., Lass, N. J., Bunnell, H. T., & Pannbacker, M. (2008). Academic and clinical training in cleft palate for speech-language pathologists. *The Cleft Palate–Craniofacial Journal, 45,* 371–380.

Vallino, L. D., Peterson-Falzone, S. J., & Napoli, J. A. (2006). The syndromes of Treacher Collins and Nager. *Advances in Speech Language Pathology, 8,* 34–44.

Vallino, L. D., Zuker, R., & Napoli, J. A. (2008). A study of speech, language, hearing, and dentition in children with cleft lip only. *The Cleft Palate–Craniofacial Journal, 45,* 485–494.

Vallino-Napoli, L. D. (2012). Evaluation and evidence-based practice. In A. Lohmander & S. Howard (Eds.), *Cleft palate speech: Assessment and intervention* (pp. 317–358). West Sussex, UK: Wiley.

Whitehill, T. L. (2002). Assessing intelligibility in speakers with cleft palate: A critical review of the literature. *The Cleft Palate–Craniofacial Journal, 39,* 50–58.

Whitehill, T. L. & Chau, C. (2004). Single-word intelligibility in speakers with repaired cleft palate. *Clinical Linguistics & Phonetics, 18,* 341–355.

Williams, A. L. (2003). *Speech disorders resource guide for preschool children*. Clifton Park, NY: Thomson Delmar Learning.

Witzel, M. A., & Vallino, L. D. (1992). Speech problems in patients with dentofacial or craniofacial deformities. *Modern Practice in Orthognathic and Reconstructive Surgery, 2,* 1687–1735.

Yorkston, K. M., Beukelman, D. R., Strand, E. A., & Hakel, M. (2010). *Management of motor speech disorders in children and adults.* Austin, TX: Pro-Ed.

Young, N. K. (2000). *TIP 38: Integrating substance abuse treatment and vocational services: Treatment Improvement Protocol (TIP) Series 38.* U.S. Department of Health and Human Services.Rockville, MD.

Zajac, D. J. (2015). The nature of nasal fricatives: Articulatory-perceptual characteristics and etiologic considerations. *SIG 5 Perspectives on Speech Science and Orofacial Disorders, 25,* 17–28.

Zajac, D. J., Cevidanes, L., Shah, S. I., & Haley, L. L. (2012). Maxillary arch dimensions and spectral characteristics with cleft lip and palate who produce middorsum palatal stops. *Journal of Speech Language and Hearing Research, 28,* 1876–1886.

Zajac, D. J. & Eshghi, M. (2017). Vocal loudness as contributory to the occurrence of obligatory posterior nasal turbulence. *The Cleft Palate-Craniofacial Journal, 55,* 301–306.

Zajac, D. J., & Preisser, J. (2016). Age and phonetic influences on velar flutter as a component of nasal turbulence in children with repaired cleft palate. *The Cleft Palate–Craniofacial Journal, 53,* 649–656.

Zajac, D. J., & Vallino, L. D. (2017). *Evaluation and management of cleft lip and palate: A developmental perspective.* San Diego, CA: Plural.

Zeiss, A. M., & Steffen, A. M. (1996). Interdisciplinary health care teams: The basic unit of geriatric care. In L. L. Carstensen, B. A. Edelstein, & L. Dornbrand (Eds.), *The practical handbook of clinical gerontology* (pp. 423–449). Thousand Oaks, CA: Sage.

Zemlin, W. R. (1998). *Speech and hearing science: Anatomy and physiology* (4th ed.). London, UK: Pearson.

■ Index

Note: Page numbers in **bold** reference non-text material.